LAURA I

Nailing Jelly

A Memoir

ANOTHER SMALL PRESS
No.3

ISBN 978-0-9957127-3-7

Published in Great Britain by Another Small Press, 2024

www.anothersmallpress.net
Cover design by Fine Fine Lines

Laura Lee Dove lives in the East Midlands. She has written fiction, poetry, flash and articles but never anticipated events in her own life would result in publishing her first book.

To all those in reality and the ether who have helped and supported me in troubled times and in the birth of this book.

Devil In Disguise

June 2016

At the age of sixty-five I have decided I was born to be a psychopath. I have no clue how or why I've come to this conclusion but feel pretty certain I am capable of heinous crimes. Although I consciously know it's a ridiculous theory, I feel terrified; both of the idea and my own state of mind. I sit on the hard, cold floor locked inside the bathroom area I share with three other patients in this hell hole. There's an incongruous sparkle in the drab, grey floor covering which always seems out of place, yet I frequently stare at it while my thoughts turn somersaults. The long mirror on the opposite wall reflects the person I used to be, but my mind belongs to someone different; someone dangerous, out of control and obsessed with destruction.

I can hear the voices of nurses outside, pretending they're looking for me, pretending they aren't aware where I am, pretending they care. I know there is little point attempting to hide or escape, but I just need someone to do something, though I have no clue what. Neither do they I suspect.

For days now I've tried to convince them I need sectioning or taking somewhere I can do no harm, where someone will know how to help me. What difference it would make I don't know; in truth I guess I just want to get away from myself and my obsessive, crazy thoughts.

Earlier this afternoon I tried various methods to convince them there is something radically wrong with me. The dinner was late arriving and patients were becoming restless and irritable as a result. I didn't care, as food repulses me, and I have to struggle to eat anything at all, but the waiting was intolerable. I believed it was somehow my fault things were delayed, eventually escaping in tears. I hate the dining room, the stale smell of revolting dinners and unwashed inmates. I hate mixing with anyone or even being seen, as I'm convinced they all despise me and are scared of the evil I feel certain emanates from my every pore. Even a short trip to the kitchen to refill my water jug has become a massive ordeal, as I know they are all watching me, judging, stepping out of my way as fear of my depraved mental state poisons the atmosphere around them.

In desperation I'd emulated the behaviour of patients I know are suffering from other severe mental health problems. Conditions I neither understand or relate to, but I know they are monitored and controlled much more than myself. But it seems no one takes me seriously, staff only smirking behind their hands or offering placebos as a way to calm me down and stop bothering them.

I'm persuaded to leave the bathroom and handed another fake tablet. I give up trying to make them understand or take any action but know my unhinged mind has to be occupied in order to prevent any more outbursts. I stay on my bed, only moving when forced or out of necessity. I frequently gaze upwards into the corner where the curtains round the bed meet, as if some divine intervention or miraculous solutions are to be found there. My mind has been searching for answers to my many problems for months, but now the problems have taken on a much more insular, intense and sinister form.

I don't know how it begins, but my distraught mind starts to inwardly repeat sequences of words backwards. This convinces me I'm being controlled by the devil, or even worse, I have taken on the role myself. For days and nights any other thoughts entering my head are dismissed as I fight to focus on turning every word I can think of backwards. I fall asleep and wake with the patterns of words repeating in my brain, dreading the endless days in between. Visitors interrupt the process, but nothing and no one can convince me I'm not the most monstrous being alive.

Sundays on the ward are particularly unbearable, with no activity, predictable, inedible meals and very little input from staff. By Sunday afternoon I realise my control over repeating backward words is diminishing. As my ability to turn words around shrinks, I become more and more perturbed, not knowing what I'm going to do with my thoughts once the words dry up completely. Eventually, I crawl into the far corner on my bed, my back against the wall and I scream; several times. It's a shock to hear this alien sound; I don't think I've ever screamed in my life, not even at Beatles' concerts in the sixties, being more prone to emotional, tearful outbursts rather than making loud noises. I know I can't continue to scream, yet feel only screaming will stop whatever demonic power is attempting to take over my mind. Eventually, two nurses come to my bedside; one bearing a cup of tea I can't hold never mind drink, the other proffering a glossy magazine as a distraction. They listen and chat for a short while, but I recognise the despair in their eyes and sense they have no idea what to do.

After they leave my only concern is finding something to distract my brain; something internal that won't draw attention to myself or disturb others. For the next few days I make words from the letters on the boards above patients' beds which contain information of their names and those of doctors and nurses. When that task is exhausted I mentally make A to Z lists of animals, places, musicians and professions until I can stand it no longer. My love of music has been starved for months, so the next diversion involves attempting to internally sing as many songs as I can. I'm devastated to realise I cannot remember much at all, perversely only recalling lyrics of songs I hate and the odd, usually disturbing line from others I barely know. I can't even remember all the words of the Lord's Prayer. To the outsider it must look like I'm doing nothing, probably in some sort of drug induced stupor, but attempting to keep my mind from being taken over by whatever force I'm petrified of is one of the hardest things I've ever had to do.

I had been admitted to the ward with severe depression and I'm painfully aware of the reasons why. After a couple of months this bizarre and terrifying state has taken over my mind and there seems no explanation. I have no control over my thoughts or emotions but feel bitterly ashamed of this hostile loathing which envelops me like some hideous, mythical creature.

I feel too distraught and ashamed to communicate with anyone. I turn off my phone to avoid any calls or texts. Staff constantly remark how lucky I am to be so cared about as they hand over cards from concerned friends all over the world. Most remain unopened. Nurses remind me I have more visitors than the rest of the ward put together, but this only increases my self hatred and guilt. All these visitors persist in attempting to console, understand and assure me I am not evil and will recover. But nothing can convince me and I find myself dreading visiting times, as being unable to think or talk of anything but my own dark thoughts fills me with self loathing.

Days pass by; the visitors refuse to desert me, but I'm acutely aware any time soon my son will be visiting me for the first time after being away on a family holiday, and this generates fresh waves of sheer terror. Despite my twisted state of mind the irony of the situation doesn't escape me. The first time he'd been in Asia I'd wanted to forcibly drag him away, but this time I'm dreading his return. I'm certain my son, a fully qualified criminologist, will despise and abandon me when he discovers the truth about his mother, the psychopath. Torture twists my insides every time I dwell on the thought he'll hate me and I'll never see my grandchildren again. But I know there is no way I'll be able to postpone his visit and cower like a fox pursued by hounds as the clock hands approach each visiting time.

Leaving On A Jet Plane

September 2006

I was born at three minutes to midnight and conclude that is one reason I am not, and never will be a morning person. Some mornings are worse than others of course, but this one has to be amongst the most miserable ever. I'm in a strange bed, I have a stinking cold and the added joy of a self induced hangover. I can hear my husband pottering around the hotel room, the familiar morning throat clearing and nose blowing adding to my desire to crawl under the duvet and stay there.

'Are you awake? Hurry up or we'll be too late for breakfast.' Even in the midst of trauma my husband's mind can still focus on his stomach. Men not only escape the inconvenience of pregnancy and the pain of childbirth, they also never experience the feelings a mother suffers when her child flies the nest. I concluded a long time ago umbilical cords have a lot to answer for.

'I can't cope with this,' I state flatly, aware the sympathy I crave won't be forthcoming.

'Of course you can. Get a move on.' It takes a mammoth effort to remove my sorry self from the bed to wash and dress. I trail behind my husband into the hotel lift, another bucket of tears threatening to ruin the small amount of make up I've managed to apply to my blotchy, drawn face. That last bottle of wine the night before had seemed a good idea at the time, but now I swear to myself I'll never drink again. Like a lot of things in my life I know it will be an empty promise and I'm the first to admit it.

'Here, blow your nose and stop crying.' He thrusts a crumpled tissue none too gently into my hand. 'You don't want people to see you snivelling.' I realise the word "people" refers to a certain couple we'd only met for the first time the previous evening.

'Well, it's not so bad for them,' I snap. 'They've got other kids, and anyway, they're snotty Southerners who think they know it all. I don't like them.' I know I'm being peevish and unfair, but I need to vent my anger and heartbreak at someone. Anyone and everyone if I'm honest.

The hotel restaurant is bustling, the smell of fried bacon, toast and coffee making me want to retch, had I enough energy. People of all nationalities and cultures queue for food or sit reading newspapers as if it's just an ordinary day.

But for me this is the day I've been dreading for months. On the whole it hasn't been a bad year compared to most. I've lost weight, joined a gym, enjoyed some great days out but knowing my only son would be leaving home in September to go travelling with a friend has taken the edge off everything. And now that day is here and I have no strategy or skills to deal with it.

Admittedly he's twenty-five now; a gentle giant with a sweet face and a heart to match, but the only time he's spent away from home has been his final year at university and that was within driving distance. But today, he's about to board a plane taking him to the other side of the world and I'm struggling to see him as an adult and not my angelic, curly haired little boy.

Heathrow airport is an impersonal, manic place, predominantly grey and unfriendly. I can see his flight to Hong Kong on the departure board is on time; any hopes of a cancellation or at least a late flight now dashed. I pretend my sodden tissues are down to the streaming cold I have but doubt I'm fooling anyone. I hand him a card to carry reminding him how much he's loved, then steal a final hug. I try to imprint the picture of his smile on my brain as he slips behind the security gates and disappears. For how long I have no idea, but I know the ache in my heart will be with me until he comes back.

We return to the car for the long drive back to our home. I'm already dreading walking through the front door knowing our son won't be there. My husband has to stop for food and the toilet of course; predictable behaviour for a practical man who tends to see everything in black and white.

'What's the matter?' he asks between munches of sandwich. Anyone with an ounce of sensitivity wouldn't need to ask. I can't put into words my feelings and know it would be a wasted effort anyway, as he'd never understand.

'I'll miss him,' is all I can manage, but even those words bring on a fresh batch of tears.

'Well, so will I,' he retorts. 'But you encouraged him. I didn't want him to go travelling in the first place, but you never tried to dissuade him.' As usual it's my fault; everything always is. Truth be known he probably blames me for the war in Afghanistan and England getting knocked out of the World Cup.

We drive home mostly in sullen silence; motorways and heavy traffic just a blur as I attempt to hold back the floodgates. Of course I'm aware he'll miss him, but he'll be more concerned about his health, his finances, his safety and more pragmatic matters. Admittedly there's some truth in his accusation; I would never stand in the way of our son's travel plans for reasons my husband and many others would never comprehend, but that doesn't make it any easier to accept.

You see, I was born in America. My father was an air force mechanic from St Louis, Missouri, stationed at Kimbolton in Cambridgeshire during World War Two. He met my mother one Saturday night in Nottingham and the rest is history as they say.

I often blame Hitler for my birth. Had it not been for the war, neither my sister or I would exist. Being a G.I. bride sounds so romantic, but a shotgun wedding in England towards the end of the world conflict was only the start of their own personal one. Even as a small child I'd picked up on their dysfunctional relationship and the chilly atmosphere being together often created.

My sister was born in England shortly after the war, but once our father was discharged the family set sail for America to start a new life. That's where mine began, along with the home sickness and resentment simmering in our mother. My sister has vague memories of life in Missouri; I have nothing but grainy old photographs and anecdotes told from the viewpoints of parents from different planets. A year after my birth I suspect my mother issued an ultimatum and the family sailed over the Atlantic again to settle in England.

For whatever reason there has always been a melancholic streak somewhere in my psyche which deprives me of contentment. I analyse the reasons, but one thing I ponder is if having an American father, yet never really being part of my family or life in the States could be a factor.

I guess racism was around in the fifties but certainly not where we lived in England. No one spoke a foreign language or had an accent other than the one associated with Nottingham. Most people were born, lived and died in the same area. So when I used to tell my friends at school that I was American, no one ever believed me. America was a different universe we only saw on Saturday mornings at the cinema, populated by cowboys and Indians and glamorous blondes. I was no different to the other children in appearance or speech, yet I often felt distanced in a way I couldn't yet comprehend.

My sister remembers being teased at school in England because of her American accent and limited knowledge due to being involved in play at kindergarten rather than the reading, writing and arithmetic curriculum of English schools. As adults we have spent many hours discussing the fact our formative years were totally different experiences, unlike most siblings. Hers spent in St Louis surrounded by our father's family and friends, mine in a poor area of Nottingham, England living in a crowded home with maternal grandparents. She has never felt the loss or burning desire to feel part of the American link as I have.

There was no opportunity to visit the States in my era. My family never returned or discussed it in full detail and I was left confused and wondering about this other half of my heritage. Air travel wasn't really an option until I was a young adult and even then flights to America were not routine and very expensive. At that stage I'd seen little of the world apart from flat maps in dog-eared atlases and a few package holidays in Europe.

So why would I stand in the way of my son's travel plans? Backpacking around the world is not something I would ever disapprove of and one of the reasons I encouraged my boy to grab the opportunities I never had. Though devastated by his leaving my heart sang out; do what you want to do my son, see what you want to see, go where you want to go. Follow your dreams and may they bring you the joy and satisfaction I have never truly found in life.

I Will Survive

October 2006

The house definitely feels different. Reminders of our absent son are everywhere and the list of things I miss grows longer by the day. The music blaring from his room, the empty place at the dinner table, the male debates over sport or politics, the key in the door in the early hours after a lad's night out, when I pretend I'm not waiting up worrying. Even the laundry basket intensifies this unfamiliar feeling of emptiness.

It's painful each time I come through the front door knowing our home will never be the same again. Of course we expect our kids to fly the nest, and it would be a worry if they didn't, but it's the uncertainty that makes it hard to accept. If our son had left home to get married, move in with mates or to take up employment elsewhere it would be easier I'm sure. Knowing he's out there somewhere heading into an unknown and potentially hazardous future means anxiety becomes a familiar sidekick and often anxiety leads down the perilous path to depression. I can't allow that to happen, so I know I will have to put avoidance strategies in place.

The computer becomes my lifeline, not only enabling me to keep in touch with him but to read of his travels and live vicariously through an online journal he keeps. The first few days spent in Hong Kong make for interesting and often amusing reading; his distinctive, chatty writing style the nearest thing there could be to actually talking to him in person and a comfort to his worried, emotional mother. Jet lag and culture shock are evident amongst the first few entries, alongside language, currency and digestive problems. As they travel, they note the long, hard stares of the Cantonese people who rarely witness a white person, let alone a six-foot-four British backpacker with his much shorter travelling companion. The cuisine, bars, modes of travel, ladies of the night and humidity all provide moments of confusion and anxiety, but they greet each new experience with acceptance and humour.

Travel plans rarely adhere to those on paper and research can never fully prepare us for the actual reality of foreign places. They're still vulnerable, inexperienced young men in many ways and failing to fully research their expedition, it's not until they reach Macau airport that they discover there are no flights from Hong Kong to Vietnam, which is their proposed next port of call.

I can sense the apprehension and moments of sheer panic as they make their own way across China by public transport amidst the chaos of a non-English speaking country. After a thirteen hour journey on a cattle truck of a train and a hair raising rickshaw ride, they manage to cross the border into Hanoi for the princely sum of seven pence.

There are sighs of relief on both sides of the globe, thanking the powers that be for their survival and the journal in the ether that enables us to keep body and soul together back at home. Reading of their experiences makes it easier to envisage places, imagine the circumstances and share emotions; the next best thing to actually being there. I ponder if such technology had been around when my own mother was living in America, if she would have felt less isolated and able to cope; If she'd have settled there and all our lives would have turned out totally differently. Contemplating imponderables may seem like a waste of time, but it's something I frequently indulge in, alongside speculating whether destiny, fate and karma really do exist.

My husband feels the absence I know, but he's a practical person and his rather macho personality prevents him from discussing his feelings in depth or showing what he'd consider any weaknesses. A creature of habit, he's slipped easily back into his routines. He's a bit of an insular soul, generally only needing his family, and is content in his own company. He's always found it difficult to accept I'm different, needing to socialise and enjoy the company of others. It's caused a lot of problems throughout our married life, and it seems impossible to find a solution, or even a compromise. We have some similar personality traits and he certainly has some admirable qualities, but his very worst in my mind is the green eyed monster that has been part of our married life from the start. We also have some interests in common, and most of those we don't share pose few problems. The one that has threatened to break our relationship and caused many difficult issues is technology, more specifically the "bloody internet," as he calls it. So, even though he follows the journal, he's more concerned about their finances, the practical details of their travels and whether they've changed their underwear.

I believe my generation has probably seen more dramatic changes than any other ever has or will again. Technology gets its fair share of bad publicity and, of course, as with most things there's a downside, but for me it has frequently been a life saver.

Being the victim of an analytical brain is something my doctor picked up on during a severe depressive phase in my thirties. He prescribed the purchase of a computer and it has probably helped me survive more than any medication or therapy sessions. We bought a Commodore 64 for my son's sixth birthday and quickly became hooked. I remember the days of rushing home after collecting him from school in order to load a tape of our latest obsession, be it Pac man, Popeye or a little bouncing egg called Dizzy. There was time to brew tea and start the dinner while we waited for all the stripy screens to settle down so we could proceed, but in those times instant gratification wasn't the norm, and I believe as a whole humanity was more patient. From there we advanced to an Amiga, then plunged into the mysterious world of the P.C. complete with C Drives, MS Dos and all its added complications. My sister also kept up with the progress of the technical world and I remember how in awe we felt when it was announced we'd one day be able to chat to each other via our computers.

The advent of the internet changed everything on a world wide and personal level; for me it opened up a whole new dimension, enabled some amazing experiences and has been an antidote for many dark periods. Technology may not be a cure for depression, but I believe it can be helpful therapy, particularly for putting things into perspective and reaching out to others in similar circumstances. For a generally gregarious person like myself, it has been a wonderful tool which has enabled me to make friends with people from all over the world, who have helped and supported me through many difficult times.

Unfortunately, my husband could never see it that way and it caused a lot of problems after we both retired from teaching. Beyond checking his bank balance, football and cricket results, ordering parts for his model railway making obsession and communicating with his family he sees little use for it.

'I don't need to go searching for people like you do,' he frequently sneers, as if it's a weakness or a flaw in my character.

Our differences regarding mingling with others has always caused problems, the internet making matters far worse. He's always resented any time I spend outside the home socialising, and frequently makes his disapproval clearly obvious. But once at home behind closed doors, with only phone calls or letters as means of communication with the outside world there wasn't too much disharmony. But then along came the internet. Problems started with the birth of the Friends Reunited website. I was thrilled to reconnect with most of my old school friends, both male and female. Admittedly, some were ex boyfriends but having left school almost forty years before the advent of the site I wasn't planning on rekindling any old flames or entering into any steamy affairs. I was just pleased to know they were still on the mortal coil and wanted to know how life had treated them since those long ago days of school.

Things deteriorated further when, during a depressive bout shortly after retiring, a friend suggested I join her chatroom. I was reluctant, particularly as it was a football based one and my knowledge and love of the beautiful game was decidedly limited. The friend wasn't one of my closest but a very insistent and forceful character who would not accept no for an answer. I didn't feel I wanted to chat to strangers or probably make a fool of myself, but I found myself launched into a new situation which unbeknown to me would lead to many opportunities. I discovered I rather liked the anonymity of the chatroom and my ability to make people laugh, regardless of not knowing who they were. Harmless fun in my humble opinion, and a definite distraction from my own rather dark and depressive thoughts.

My husband hated the idea I may be actually chatting online to men, concluding all who used the internet were bound to be perverts, paedophiles or psychopaths. I tried to point out to him that not exposing any identity meant anyone could be any age, gender or species they chose, and what did it matter if it offered a bit of light relief? At the time I wasn't interested in meeting any of these people but enjoyed the banter and distraction. But nothing would quell his suspicions or anger. For many of our evenings at home with him in front of his beloved television and myself on the computer, tension filled the air like winter fog and I found myself becoming more anxious every time he put me under the microscope or in the witness box. A typical evening would end up in some sort of heavy debate after being bombarded by questions from the armchair.

'What site are you on now?'

'Who are you chatting to?'

'Is your sister online?'

'What do you find to talk about?'

'Don't you think you should go to bed?'

'Why are you getting annoyed?'

This inevitably led to a full scale row which resulted in nothing, apart from him falling asleep before his head hit the pillow and me lying awake crying with the frustration and injustice of it all. Mornings often brought some sort of strangled apology but did little to change the situation.

Eventually the chatroom collapsed, alongside my friendship with the initiator. At the time I was unaware a very special, treasured friendship, worth far more than the one I'd lost would result from my time spent in that chatroom, so maybe things do happen for a reason and there's no such thing as coincidence. Online, I moved on to playing word games with people from many different countries, as well as making a multitude of firm friends on a writing website; activities far better suited to my nature and interests than football.

Some may not agree, but in a relationship with someone constantly suspicious and insanely jealous, survival means learning avoidance strategies, which include hiding anything which may be considered provocative, no matter how innocuous we consider them ourselves. Even an X at the end of an email to a friend causes disapproval and interrogation, yet he can't see how ridiculous it is to send his wife an email every day and expect a detailed reply. A sad state of affairs, but jealousy and possessiveness have played starring roles for most of my married life. I keep my emails as well hidden as I know how, my days out with old friends undercover and avoid as much conversation as possible about the group reunions I attend but frequently suffer for my sins after my husband "accidentally" accesses my emails; something he's grown to be an expert at.

At least our son's travel journal is of mutual interest and something we can openly share. The backpackers spend over six weeks travelling in Vietnam, visiting many different places and meeting many other travellers along the way. Festivals, transport, kayaking and even a typhoon are recorded in their journals along with more sinister observations regarding hard sells, including drugs and boom-boom, as it's referred to on those soils. Pickpockets, prostitutes, children selling anything they can get their hands on and poverty seem to dominate a country obsessed with money and sex, which only accentuates the relative innocence and vulnerability of two inexperienced Westerners.

On reaching the border into Cambodia it's obvious the same and worse conditions exist. Corruption is evident from the start; travellers failing to produce the necessary documents forced to pay extortionate sums to enter the country, then witnessing their money being pocketed by officials. Travelling towards Phnom Penh many shady towns and begging children are observed, alongside notices warning of child prostitution. A sinister, depraved and damaged nation still suffering from the atrocities of Pol Pot, it seems the khmer culture is so complex and inconsistent not even the khmer people themselves understand it. Our son visits most tourist attractions, including the museums and killing fields, where the horrors of torture are still clearly evident and commentaries spare none of the gory, bone chilling details. It proves a very sobering experience and I suspect they are relieved to move on to the more tranquil seaside resort of Sihanoukville.

It's then our son and his travelling companion part company, something we had advised against but are assured is perfectly safe. He takes up residence at a guest house by the beach where he's offered free accommodation, provided he eats and drinks at the family restaurant. The small room he occupies is shared with mosquitoes and cockroaches and within days he's suffering from a severe eye infection which renders him unable to travel or explore very far. He spends his time doing very little apart from socialising with the family and sleeping; his journal entries reflecting his lethargy and containing only news of his hosts.

I have no idea as I read about the heartbreak of the killing fields, that a few days later I will receive a telephone call from Cambodia which will shock me to the core on a personal level and completely alter the course of all our lives.

Everybody Hurts

November 2006

It's a chilly November morning when I settle at the computer with my first cup of tea to check my emails. I discover one from my son stating he's going to phone from Cambodia later in the morning and requests I answer the call rather than his father, as he thinks what he has to tell us will be better received by me. He adds not to worry as he considers it good news.

As I pace the floor waiting for the call, I guess I already suspect what the announcement is going to be. What else would an innocent young man regard as good news for his mother to hear other than wedding plans? But my confusion over who the chosen bride can be rings loud bells of alarm. As far as I'm aware his travel plans are on hold while he recovers from an infection and the only people he's associating with are the owners of the guest house he's staying at. I know they have a gaggle of daughters, one of them disabled with a newborn baby, who my son has mentioned several times in his travel blog. Surely not?

My worst fears are confirmed when we speak. I don't handle the call or the news well, devastation robbing me of any coherent words or reasoning. How can my son, the brightest, most caring and popular of young men possibly be contemplating marriage to someone he has only known a matter of days? How can he not envisage the problems he'll have to face with a foreign, disabled partner? How can he think for a minute he'll be able to cope with a wife and someone else's baby into the bargain? Questions and concerns bombard my brain and everything else takes a back seat as I wrestle with emotions that threaten to drown any sensible meaning life has ever held.

My husband reacts in his usual subtle way by sending an email worded "Come home you fucking idiot," then threatens to pack a case and fly out to Cambodia. I know from experience that's just another idle threat. Fear of losing control has been his lifelong phobia, but in this situation neither of us hold any power and I try to convince him we must work together from the same page, hoping against hope some unity will ensue and at least delay our son's rash decision.

Over the next few days there are phone calls, e-mails and much time spent desperately seeking answers as to what we can do. Two months of travelling in unfamiliar and often deprived areas, observing tragedy and being unwell convinces me he isn't thinking straight. What can I say to a son who thinks he's in love and can't understand why I can't support his plans? This is the son who didn't want to settle down, intended seeing the world and doing so many things. I loved him for that. What can I do to stop him making the biggest mistake of his life? His future held so much promise. Now he has chosen to take on a woman from an alien culture with much baggage and cannot see why his parents are devastated. He's an innocent, a soft hearted soul, a lovely person, but I want to scream at him not to do this. He plans on marrying in January and bringing her back to England soon after. I will never cast him aside, but if he goes ahead with this I know it will be one of the hardest things I've ever had to come to terms with.

We watch the horror on the faces of family and friends as we relay our son's plans, taking small comfort from them we are not overreacting. Everyone concerned sends messages via the internet asking him to stop and think about his proposed actions, delay his plans, keep travelling then return to Cambodia if he still feels the same, bring the girl home for us to meet before making any commitments. Like a cornered rat, he retreats, and having the upper hand as regards communication offers little response, only relaying how hurt he and his intended feel by our lack of support. I know even now nothing will stop this wedding.

For days I walk around in a daze waiting for the moment I'll wake up from this nightmare. But every morning I am faced with the knowledge this is no bizarre dream but a reality no parent could possibly have anticipated. My head whirls constantly with anxiety and the fear depression will soon take over. The familiar symptoms kick in; the inability to eat, sleep or concentrate and I know I cannot allow myself to sink into the pit or I will be no use to anyone and that would be an impossible situation.

Obsessional thinking often accompanies the mind of a depressive. It's not necessarily a problem and can even be an advantage when the thinking is positive or productive. But in negative circumstances or times of massive anxiety it becomes the enemy, feeding itself and spiralling out of control, a runaway vehicle freewheeling to its inevitable fate. It doesn't take long before the sufferer becomes a complete mental wreck and unable to function even at a basic level. I teeter on the edge of the depression abyss, the familiar black tentacles beckoning more intensely as days pass by in a murky haze of tears, frustration and mental anguish. I have been here before and had hoped to never return to a state where the desire to live another day is annihilated.

I have a very sympathetic doctor who knows my history and seems to have some understanding of my mental condition. I do not want to take medication or end up in hospital again so my one visit to see him is enough. He confirms my reaction to the bombshell is in no way abnormal, and tries to comfort me by suggesting relationships like the one my son is planning on entering do not last and Asian girls often find it difficult to settle in England. I leave the surgery determined to somehow find my own ways of coping with the whirling thoughts and dark feelings.

Talking can be helpful therapy but tensions being so high, conversations with my husband generally result in heavy debates and very different concerns. I'm pretty sure he's communicating secretly with our son, expressing his own views and probably anticipating brownie points for disagreeing with mine. This makes me angry, as he frequently accuses me of acting deviously and keeping secrets, but this is not the time to enter into further disharmony by reopening old wounds.

My mother has always been a source of comfort and wise words in the past, but now she is suffering from dementia and would hardly be able to take the situation on board, never mind offer guidance. My father, a reserved octogenarian, has never really been involved in his daughter's emotional episodes or traumatic family circumstances. He states it will never happen, then returns to reading his newspaper. My sister lives away so her input is limited, but she and good friends do the best they can to help and console.

Again, I turn to the internet and the friends I have made through word games and writing. I do not exaggerate when I say these people help more than anything else with their sympathetic comments, their very wise advice and relaying their own family traumas which help put things into perspective. One friend asks me to consider the possibility it might all work out well and result in a happy ever after, something my negative tendencies haven't contemplated before. It seems highly unlikely but not an impossibility.

I conclude there is nothing I can do. My child is distanced, besotted and there is no way to reason through sparse communication. I bumble through each day praying for a miracle I know won't happen; my mind asking a thousand questions, querying my own parenting skills and cartwheeling through anger, despair, heartbreak and sheer terror on an hourly basis.

I cannot convey how many emotions are competing for dominance in my whirling head but know anger is the most destructive one. I'm angry for many reasons and angry at myself for being angry. I hate aggression; my mother can be aggressive, as can my husband. I've worked hard to avoid being antagonistic, considering anger a wasted emotion I don't like having. I make the conscious decision to do nothing more or have any contact with my son until the anger has lessened. For my own sake, I cannot allow negativity and anger to eat away at me or I will self-destruct and by doing so I will alienate my son. That is something I couldn't live with.

Repeatedly telling myself far worse things can happen and confident the loving relationship I have always shared with my son will not be broken or damaged in any way, I gradually find a way to ask some heartfelt questions and convey my disquiet in a more tolerant fashion. But nothing is easily expressed through e-mails, where meaning and tone can be misconstrued or through words spoken on telephones accompanied by static, distortion and delay, so much as an acceptance of sorts slowly commences, it will be an agonising few months before any of the issues and anxieties can be addressed properly. I manage to dampen the anger and fight off the threat of severe depression, but I am far from serene or emotionally stable. I've always been prone to pulling myself apart, but right now it feels like the whole world is conspiring against me.

So it is, on a cold, rainy Sunday in January our son spends the day getting married Buddhist style, thousands of miles away, to a foreign, disabled girl we have never met and know very little about. What we do know is hardly reassuring, but there is nothing to do except let it be. I have a heavy cold and remark it's a good job there's no way we could attend, as my nose would have clashed violently with the red hat I reserve for weddings. I spend the day at home, my thoughts and fears swirling like a threatening tornado, the tears refusing to abate as I imagine my son laughing and celebrating with his new bride. The nightmare I'd hoped to wake up from now a reality, the future a huge question mark hovering precariously above a fragile, bleak horizon.

Into The Unknown

January 2007

My days return to mundane routines, yet my mind is constantly occupied with the very dramatic change in our lives now we have a daughter-in-law we have yet to meet. Not something we could ever have anticipated and admittedly wouldn't have wanted, but the unpredictability of life is something I am already very familiar with. Although we have come to terms with the wedding to some extent, we have little or no idea what lies ahead and it's difficult to envisage many positives.

I can't resist fantasising about changes I'd appreciate in my own life. Things far removed from the real world and all its worries, like a lottery win, a world cruise, a sylph like figure or hubby spending an evening at the pub. They'd probably all require a miracle, but there's no harm in dreaming. In reality, I've come to dread the start of each new year, uncertainties and fear taking the place of resolutions and hope.

Predictably, I wake up in the mornings with the same old feeling, the same old urge to turn over and go back to sleep and the same old grumpy other half clanging pots in the kitchen. Many afternoons I visit my parents, where the temperature is enough to fool you you're in hell and mother's music choice enough to confirm it. Lately it's been war time warbles about white cliffs and promising to meet again some sunny day, while mother reminisces over personal memories from the era and assumes mine to be the same. I just make appropriate noises and nod of late; depending on the day, the weather or if there's an R in the month, my mother believes me to be any age ranging from ten to seventy. I try to make light of things but am only covering up the hurt I feel dealing with my demanding and stressful days. Unrelenting anxiety and depressive moods follow me everywhere, like sinister dark shadows.

My parents are an increasing worry. My mother's condition is deteriorating and she's not prepared to admit it. My father, at eighty-seven, is growing very frail, frequently suffering bad falls. They barely communicate and I am the only carer. Every day I have to think for them, organise their appointments, medicines, shopping and other needs and am becoming very weary of it all. There is no help available and I live in dread of the inevitable. My ninety-two-year old mother-in-law also needs help and has recently spent some time in hospital.

My son has been the light of my life. I've attempted to never be an overbearing mother as my own has sometimes been, and have allowed him to be his own person. Biased I may be, but I consider him a wonderful human being; warm, honest, intelligent, funny and caring. I've supported his travels whole-heartedly despite knowing it would be a wrench. It is his life and I wanted him to live it without the confines I have endured. I love him and that will never alter, but his actions are something I'm finding extremely difficult to cope with, at the same time berating myself. Other people handle challenges without crumbling, so why can't I? Why do I always seem to see things through negative eyes? I frequently conclude the only positive thing about me is my blood group.

After the wedding his travel blog entries have become sporadic and vague, his phone calls infrequent and often accompanied by static and delay. A lot of soul searching on my part occupies my thoughts. I conclude my sensitive son considers himself the proverbial knight on a white charger, rescuing what he sees as a "diamond in the rough," to use his own words from a harsh life in a corrupt country. Whether he is deluded and sucked in by circumstances is uncertain, but I'm pretty sure his experiences with women are limited and he's not been swept off his feet before. I cast my mind back to my younger days, to the times I've declared undying love; that feeling of never wanting to be parted from someone easily forgotten after many years of marriage. If I take myself back in time I can rekindle it and it helps my understanding to some extent.

Every marriage carries risks and there is no guarantee it will survive even if you have known your partner a long time before taking the plunge. My parent's marriage can hardly be described as a success and my own is far from perfect, despite knowing my husband for several years before our wedding. I had ended a long term affair with a man who was probably the love of my life to enter into this new relationship. I suspect I drifted into marriage, partly due to fear of becoming an old spinster teacher with a house full of cats and a certain amount of pressure from the groom. My husband to be, a brusque and stern teacher at the school where I also worked, whose first marriage had resulted in a cheating wife, a divorce, two dogs and custody of his four-year-old daughter convinced me things would be easier all round once we were married.

Our wedding took place on a bright and breezy August afternoon. I remember walking back from the hairdressers, my footsteps hesitating as waves of panic and uncertainty swept over me. I persuaded myself it was just a case of wedding day nerves, but I suspect I knew deep down there were other, more disturbing reasons.

It was a simple affair. A registry office agreement; divorcees not being allowed to marry in church at that time. A basic buffet for family and friends and no honeymoon due to the groom not wishing to leave his young daughter behind.

Slipping into a routine at my new home in a run down area of Nottinghamshire wasn't plain sailing. The house he'd shared with his first wife was not an ideal start in my opinion and its position isolated and impractical. But such things were not discussed, and we returned to our respective teaching jobs in September. By this time my husband had transferred to a Special Education school where he eventually became Headmaster.

Struggles with the stepdaughter came with the new role. Resentment on both sides I'll admit. Battles over meals a daily occurrence, more to do with the cook than the food. Too many temper tantrums won by the smaller contestant as guilt haunted the father and overcompensation seemed the answer to doting grandparents.

The first bout of jealous, unreasonable behaviour occurred within a few months after I'd spent a weekend in France with teaching colleagues. The return night ferry was late due to rough seas and the coach home delayed. I was met by a very angry man who seemed to blame me personally, instigating a lengthy debate and serious interrogation. This was alien behaviour to me and I was clueless as to how to deal with it, yet uncomfortably aware that lack of trust on one side and fear on the other were not the best companions for a successful relationship.

Just over a year later my time was taken up with my new baby. I'd moved from a city to live in the middle of nowhere, I'd given up my career to look after my son and it was a pretty lonely time. Later I joined a mother and toddler group to meet new people. The first Christmas all the ladies went out on a coach for a meal. When I arrived back at eleven at night I was greeted by that same angry, nasty person and suffered hours of verbal abuse as to why the coach was so late back. I told him how ridiculous he was being and received an apology of sorts the next day, but the exact same thing happened the following Christmas. I didn't enjoy the outing at all as I was nervous of what would be said on return. The other mothers found it difficult to believe my situation.

Son started school, I returned to part time work and years rolled by. I made some good friends in teaching and once in a while we'd go out for a meal or a drink. Every time I went out I returned to the same grumpy, silent treatment, followed by verbal abuse. Eventually the outings dwindled as people moved on or started families.

I used to think his insane jealousy stemmed from his first wife committing adultery but still it is not an excuse. I have never been unfaithful and have no intentions of being, yet the jealousy and controlling behaviour continues. These days, I don't think that is the root cause; I just think it's an innate part of his nature. He'd do anything for the kids and to help my family. He'd get me anything I wanted if he thought it would make me happy. He cares when I'm ill, upset or depressed. He's a big help in the home and I know he worships the ground I walk on. But that's part of the problem; I don't want to be placed on a pedestal and be someone's possession. My freedom of choice is more important and I just wish I'd thrashed this out many years ago. He's somewhat more tolerant than he used to be, but the damage is done and I cannot rid my heart of the bitter resentment at what I've endured and the things I've missed out on. I've been made to feel on trial and found guilty for things that ordinary people do all the time without any hassle.

I didn't see any of this coming when I married him and feel it's important for any couple to be extremely careful before making any commitment. So, is it any wonder I have little faith in the marriage my son has entered into? I still believe he'll have many problems to deal with and is making a huge mistake. I cannot deny there are many times I feel he is being used as a meal ticket and a means of escape for a very desperate young lady. The future for us all is unknown, and I am very aware unanticipated events can wreak havoc with our lives. What exactly we will be facing is almost impossible to contemplate, but I have a feeling none of it will be straightforward.

Love Changes Everything

March 2007

No matter how long people have been a part of our lives I wonder if we ever really know or understand them. Can we ever say that someone is totally predictable? Do we even fully know ourselves? Over the years I have probably been pleasantly surprised and deeply shocked by everyone in my life, including my nearest and dearest. I could never have anticipated my son would present me with the biggest shock of all, and I have to confess I feel deeply disappointed in the road he has chosen. But my love for him means I have to learn to look at things from different angles, accept no one can accurately predict the future and maybe there's even a chance it will all turn out well. I am trying to be tolerant and open minded but it's difficult to imagine our future path will be a smooth one.

It's also obvious there is much we do not know about our new daughter-in-law, or her background, her life and culture. I am spending a lot of time researching the Khmer way of life, the beliefs, history and social interaction. My husband reminds me a little knowledge is a dangerous thing, but I'm not going to opt for ignorance as I believe it will be far from bliss. I find my research interesting, confusing, reassuring in some ways yet terrifying in others, and of course I don't believe everything I discover to be the absolute truth.

The golden age of Cambodia was between the ninth and fourteenth century, during the Angkor period, which was a powerful and prosperous empire that had flourished and dominated almost all of inland Southeast Asia. The horrors of the Khmer Rouge will certainly never be forgotten and scars will be carried for generations, but according to research, faced with any challenge Cambodians have the innate ability to pick themselves up, dust themselves down and carry on. Respect supposedly plays a huge role in Cambodian society as elders are held in high regard, and with no social support system children are expected to provide for their parents as they grow older.

I read of the traits ingrained in Cambodians. Their gentle nature, kindness, caring attitudes and the ability to face everything wearing a smile. As a deeply Buddhist country the philosophy of being thoughtful and compassionate forms part of daily life in Cambodia.

I have never been a fan of organised religion, but Buddhism has always appealed to me on many levels. My mother has always been a devout Spiritualist and I have accompanied her to many services in the past, so I know the two faiths bear similarities. I am not an unwavering believer but find the principles of Spiritualism intriguing, and have to admit I've seen some pretty impressive demonstrations by Mediums.

I find some comfort in the positive aspects of my research, but there is a much darker side to this country and its culture, particularly where Cambodian women are concerned.

Traditionally, Cambodian girls are compared to a piece of cotton wool and boys to a diamond. A diamond, when dropped into mud can be washed as clean and sparkling as before, while cotton wool can never regain its purity once it has been dirtied. In conventional Cambodian society arranged marriages are the norm, divorce is taboo and international marriages rare. Girls who engage in premarital sex are supposedly considered beyond redemption.

Conversely, it seems in present times the sex trade in Cambodia is not only alive and well, but flourishing. Girls as young as twelve and thirteen are being trafficked into the system as a way of earning collateral for their family's debts. Virgins bring in the most money and many young girls are tricked by family into joining the ranks of prostitution before they are even aware of their own sexuality. It's chilling to read of thousands of underage girls being sold into sexual slavery and to think there are over a hundred thousand prostitutes under the age of eighteen. Visitors to Cambodia may be impressed by how upbeat and modern parts of this country appear to be but still thirty-five per cent of Cambodians earn less than thirty pence a day and live in abject poverty. With little employment or education, families soon find themselves in debt and it seems the easiest way to earn money is to allow or sell your beautiful, young female relatives to work for pimps and brothels.

Girls as young as twelve are reportedly beaten, stabbed, drugged, raped and threatened at gunpoint every night in what is considered their work. Further research leads me to believe in certain brothels and for the right price, even four-year-old girls can be used as sexual playthings for the depraved and perverted clients.

All this is alarming enough, but add the unwanted pregnancies, the sexually transmitted diseases and one of the highest incidents of AIDS in the world to the equation and it becomes even more so.

Beer gardens, massage parlours and karaoke bars are all legal and swarming with stunning young girls awaiting customers, many looking and acting far older than their actual tender years. My son has witnessed and condemned such places, which adds more jagged pieces to this bewildering puzzle.

What are we to make of our new Cambodian daughter-in-law? Apart from the information our son has provided us with and some wedding photographs, we have no way of forming an accurate impression. We know she was hit by a train as a toddler, leading to the amputation of her right arm and that she's the only one of the six children in her family to speak English. We learn she's already left Cambodia once at the age of seventeen to live with a man in Germany who'd promised her the earth then proceeded to abuse and mistreat her until she fled and returned home. We also know the father of her baby girl is an English man who obviously did not hang around once her pregnancy was confirmed. We also discover both her parents are confirmed as H.I.V. positive but continue to work and run a restaurant in Sihanoukville. It seems possible their disabled daughter is a pawn they've used to draw customers into the restaurant, as well as helping with cooking and waiting tables.

Always the practical one in our relationship, my husband tends to see things in monochrome and I suspect he suffers from ostrich syndrome when it comes to potential problematic situations. Although very concerned, he continues to get on with life and it's probably a good thing he is not the emotional wreck I am transforming into. Anything for family and exclude the rest of the world is his mantra. I contemplate how he'll feel when his kitchen sink is invaded, the washing basket is overflowing, his vacuum cleaner and ironing board are abducted, alien aromas drift from the kitchen and his comfortable routine is disrupted, but I keep these thoughts to myself.

It's time for me to put into practice some of the platitudes I have carelessly thrown at others over the years. I have no problems with race or disability but am aware culture differences on both sides may not be easy to overcome. It's difficult, yet necessary, to reserve judgement and not question the values or beliefs of a culture we know little about. Neither can I allow myself to judge my son's wife indiscriminately. Walking that mile in someone else's shoes is a philosophy I try to cling to, for we are all victims of the circumstances we find ourselves living in. None of this comes easily.

We reassure our son we'll do our best to welcome his new wife and make her feel as comfortable as possible should they decide to return to England. However, we make it clear we cannot entertain having a baby living with us, which doesn't seem to go down too well. We are informed they've decided to do a little touring in Cambodia before heading to Australia in February, where they intend to find work and save some funds before returning to England. Their plans seem to be changing more often than their underwear I suspect, and it all sounds rather idealistic to my cynical head, but we all learn through trial and error and we have to allow our son to make his own decisions from now on.

As predicted, problems abound as they discover Australian authorities will only allow his new wife a three-month visa and the baby declared too young to enter the country. My alarm at the altered plan to leave baby behind has to be suppressed and allowances made for a culture where the extended family is dominant and it isn't so unusual for family to care for children while mothers work or fulfil other plans. However, remembering how much time I'd invested in my son as a baby and how devastating it would have been to leave him for months make it difficult to accept their decision.

In Australia they stay with a friend and my son finds menial work for a while, but it's obvious the optimistic plans they had are not materialising and by May they are on their way to England, minus the child. We know it's going to be a strain having a young couple living with us, particularly as one is a total stranger, unfamiliar with our country and disabled into the bargain. Some parents may have washed their hands of the whole situation, others might have hardened themselves to tell them to support themselves, but rightly or wrongly we feel we can't do that, so have to brace ourselves for a complete change to our lives and offer support in order to give them a chance at making a success of life here.

My involvement with the online writing site continues to bring a lot of comfort and my reader's support helps tremendously, enabling me to see this isn't the end of the world but possibly an opportunity to build bridges and face the future with hope. As the newlyweds make their way back to England one member in Singapore provides them with free accommodation complete with pool, gym, sauna and maid. The world is certainly a smaller place thanks to the internet and the kindness of strangers enough to restore some of my faith.

In early May we spend a restless night at a hotel near Gatwick airport where the couple's plane will land the next day. Nerves and anxiety mingle with the anticipation of seeing our son for the first time in almost a year and the mystery of meeting his wife.

The flight is due to land around six in the morning and we will try to put the past behind us and begin a new phase with our son and the daughter-in-law we will meet for the first time. It is pointless to dwell on what the future holds for too long. Although I have mixed emotions and fears, I feel determined to try and make the best of it. Turning a negative into a positive is a possibility and a much more pleasant feeling to live with. The time leading up to this moment has been an emotional rollercoaster fuelled by anxiety and tears, but one thing is certain. Despite sparse communication, we have established we are still the same people as before he left, our relationship will not be ruined whatever happens and we can work this through. Love changes everything.

Under Pressure

May 2007

He hadn't told us about the leg. It would be the first of many omissions, half truths and deceptions, but right now we have no idea what lies ahead. Even thinking about it is too painful and frightening.

Five minutes ago we watched our only son emerge from the arrivals at Gatwick airport's north terminal. Emotions ran high, just as they had nine months earlier at Heathrow as we'd watched him leave. How many emotions are there? In less than a year I think I've experienced most of them, though sadly more negative than positive.

He looks well. He's gained some weight and his time in the sun has turned his normally pale skin an attractive shade of gold. I can't wait to hug him; my precious boy, my only child, my opus magnum. My heavy heart, almost shattered to pieces by actions from the previous months, lifts slightly as he walks towards us with that familiar, cheeky grin.

But confusion joins the ranks as I look around for his partner. Although I only have eyes for him, I can't fail to notice he's distinctly alone. Dare I hope he's changed his plans, backed out at the last minute and ended the nightmare we've endured for what seems like eternity?

After wiping away the tears of relief, mixed with the familiar ones of turmoil and anxiety I gaze into the eyes of this boy I thought I'd known inside out, now twenty-five years old and towering over me. Not a boy at all, but a mother's eyes refuse to see their children as independent adults. I know in that moment I will never stop loving him no matter what he's done or what lies ahead.

'Where is she?' I ask tentatively, hoping my tone reflects none of my inner feelings.

'She'll be here soon,' he replies. 'She can't walk far so someone is bringing her in a wheelchair.'

I ask no further questions despite the new ones adding themselves to my already overloaded brain.

We help him carry his bags to the airport exit and there she is. I recognise her from photographs I've seen but realise they have disguised many things. She's shorter and dumpier than I'd imagined and not as pretty as many pictures have portrayed her. Her clothes are cheap, ill matched and unflattering, but thankfully the scarf she wears conceals the missing limb, though it's a hard fact to disregard, despite not being visible.

Her smile is discerning and rather beautiful, revealing even white teeth I can only envy, framed by full, rosy lips. I return her smile and hold out my arms to welcome her.

'You look just like your Mum,' she states excitedly, her grin spreading as she looks first at our son and then at us. Her voice is loud, rather shrill and her broken English evident. She continues to chatter, already confirming she's no demure, subservient creature, which is disappointing and reassuring at the same time.

'How far away is the car?' asks our son as we turn towards the road.

'Not far,' I reply. 'You know your Dad can't walk too well these days so it's parked in a disabled spot.'

I resist asking why it matters, but it soon becomes perfectly clear. I try not to stare at the wasted leg, the ill fitting shoe and the clumsy gait of this newcomer as we walk towards the car park. He should have told us about the leg.

The drive home is hardly relaxing, but conversation flows and it's obvious whatever adjectives will arise to describe our new daughter-in-law, shy isn't one of them. Her first observation is the unwillingness of passing drivers to return waves and smiles, followed by negative comments about the weather and unfamiliar landscapes. A niggle is already forming; how on earth will this woman cope in a country so far removed from her own, in distance, climate and lifestyle?

If I imagined travelling or marriage would dramatically change my son, then I am initially mistaken. He still seems the same easy going, clumsy and amusing young man I remember. The only difference I witness is the addition of a pair of rose-coloured spectacles. Obviously, future life for him and us has certainly altered and we all know the next few months will be a testing time. His wife has a six month visa and the plan is to see if she likes England, in which case they'll return to Cambodia and bring baby back with them. If not, then who knows?

Wanting to start out on the right foot, I've placed many welcome home gifts in what is to be their room and we've decided for the first evening we'll take the couple out for a meal of their choice. It's obvious from the start his wife is not afraid to voice her opinions or express her preferences. It's May, the weather is unseasonably cold and gloomy, and once we've arrived back at our house she's soon tucked under a blanket and fast asleep on the sofa. We put it down to jet lag and send out for food later.

Over the next few weeks we see many sides to her character and use an abundance of adjectives in an effort to describe her, but an enigma probably fits best. One day she's cheerful, helpful, friendly and loving, another she's sullen, lazy, disgruntled and demanding. It's not easy to accept or adjust to the invasion of weird vegetables with appendages, rice steamers, strange cooking aromas, phone calls from Asian friends and relatives who speak little English, and Khmer music or films running constantly on computers.

Neither is it easy for her to adjust to our climate or culture. She finds it difficult to adapt to our unpredictable and often miserable weather or understand why shops and restaurants don't supply the food she prefers. She tells us of poor families in Cambodia serving up the next door's deceased dog for dinner, yet frequently leaves English dishes uneaten. She declares British people are grumpy and unfriendly and maybe she's correct in her conclusion it's our weather that's responsible. But her biggest problem is her inability to accept the small families here who do not live under one roof or interact on a daily basis.

She seems to have read her favourite story of Cinderella too frequently and I suspect the impression she's formed of life in the West is far from the reality. She talks constantly of her life in Cambodia and it's obvious the values of a nation obsessed by money, appearance, sex and food are not going to disappear from her agenda.

Sometimes it's easy to observe the qualities our son has been charmed by. Innately intelligent and observant, strong-spirited and determined, talented and capable despite her disabilities are all admirable traits. Despite her limited English and strong accent she can be extremely funny and her openness at times refreshing and engaging. She christens my husband Mr Bean and refers to our son as Big Boy and there are many occasions when laughter prevails.

However, there's a darker side to her character I recognise fairly early on; maybe a case of it takes one to know one. Some of the revelations from her past are very disturbing, shocking even to the broadest of minds, and obviously have left mental along with physical scars. Determined not to judge, we attempt to make life for her here as comfortable as possible. Buttoning your lips when your furniture is damaged, your kitchen left looking like a disaster area, your laundry basket constantly overflowing and your time eaten up by requests for help means inside pressure builds to the point where you fear self combustion.

Our son has to find temporary work so is out most of the day and with his wife's physical disabilities it's difficult for her to go anywhere. I've given up driving so it means spending many hours in each other's company. My husband and I are also caring for three elderly and fragile parents and all in all it's a very surreal and stressful time. We take the whole family out on her twenty-first birthday in June and later hold a party in her honour. She's always happiest when the centre of attention, but friends and family are starting to see a rather over demanding, ungrateful and spiteful side to her character.

By August it becomes more obvious whatever we do or say, she's not particularly happy and I start to notice more friction between her and my son. He seems distracted, tense and unsettled, but we assume it's just a case of feeling the pressure of work, officialdom and organising plans for their return to Cambodia sometime in the near future. He assures us his feelings for his wife have not altered and her sombre moods mainly due to missing her baby and family. They decide to return to Cambodia and come back with the baby as soon as funds allow.

However, when our son loses his job for what he tells us is due to inappropriate use of the computer at work, alarm bells start to ring once more. This is so out of character and unexpected we have to question what exactly is going on. He assures us he's merely been perusing flights and playing a few games in his spare time, and as it's only temporary employment it's no big deal, so not to worry.

In late August after I've returned from a weekend away with a friend, the truth finally comes out. I'm upstairs when I hear my son crying and his wife speaking sharply, yet uncharacteristically quietly. My mind goes into overdrive pondering the possibilities when they both appear at the doorway of my room.

'Mum, I need to talk to you but please don't go mad.' He looks nervous, yet defensive at the same time. Is she pregnant? Are they parting? Do they need to return to Cambodia? I have little idea what's going to be revealed but am certain it's only going to add more strain to an already tense situation.

'I'm in a mess with money,' That doesn't really surprise me but the response I receive when I ask why goes beyond a shock.

'I've been gambling on the internet, I lost all my winnings and I'm in deep debt after trying to win it back.'

In some ways it's a compliment of sorts that our son always seeks me out when he has troubles, rather than his father, and I can understand the reasons why to some extent. On this occasion I wish he'd approached him first. The fine line I've been walking on snaps, the proverbial hits the fan and some very harsh words are spoken. I may be wrong but I can only believe my son would do such a thing because of the immense pressure she is putting him under to return to Cambodia and I lash out at them both.

It's just too much for me to take on board after all we've been through but it only succeeds in making matters a lot worse. A war of words continues into the early hours and they leave the next day to spend their last few weeks with my stepdaughter and her family. It seems I'm considered public enemy number one by everyone as a result of my outburst. There are times in our lives when we wish we could retract things we've said or alter the way we've reacted and this will always be one of mine.

Everyone seems unaware how stressful things have been for me too, how I'm barely holding things together and feel everything is falling apart. I feel like I'm walking an endless tight-rope, exhausted, just waiting for the inevitable slip that will send me plummeting into the blackness below. In order to avoid that I have bottled it all up, consumed by guilt, telling myself I must think of others, help them out and never let on how low I am sinking. I guess there had to come a time when I couldn't contain it any longer, but I so wish it hadn't been now.

There follows a very painful, strained and difficult time as we attempt to build bridges. When I've calmed down somewhat I resolve we must all get through this somehow. Life is too short to forever hold grudges or become estranged from loved ones. If that ever happens I know I'll hurt more than anyone and bearing in mind our son has never caused us any problems in his toddler or teenage years, I conclude we were due for some trouble and we've hit it big time. I have always had low self esteem and I'm good at tearing myself apart, so inevitably question my own parenting skills, concluding I must be partly to blame.

On the eve of their departure to Cambodia we've patched things up enough to spend time with them at our house.

We've helped our son to sort out how he'll repay his debts and he promises to never do anything so irresponsible again. I fear I will never trust either of them completely but don't want their future impeded by negativity or ill feeling. His wife is quiet, sullen and obviously more than ready to return to her country. I dare not think about the future too much but am prepared to accept whatever decision they make about where to settle.

As they stand to leave she suddenly bursts into a torrent of tears and flies into my arms.

'Mum, I just want everything to be all right and for us all to get on,' she sobs. Knowing enough about her by this stage to recognise such an action wouldn't come easily to her, I confess my heart softens and my own tears join hers.

It will be another few months before we'll see them again, with many concerns and worrying events along the way, but at least the olive branch of forgiveness lies precariously between us.

Starting Over

November 2007

Now our son and his wife have returned to Cambodia the humdrum routines of caring for parents and regular activities have resumed. Considering the pressure and stresses of the last few months it's something of a relief but rarely are the worries and concerns about our son's situation far from my mind. The debts, the irresponsible gambling, his wife's moodiness and desire to return to Cambodia all hint that things are floundering in their relationship and the future is looking shaky. Although we've been assured they will return to England in a few months with her baby, I'm not convinced it will happen and fear of the unknown accompanies me everywhere, every day.

We have witnessed a lot of disturbing incidents ourselves and are bound to question the future. Our son has distanced himself from his own friends during their stay here, yet has driven to many places around England in order to meet Asian families his wife has discovered through the internet. Mostly strangers, but it appears her need to connect with them reflects a rather insular attitude and a desire to be the centre of attention. Inevitably the relationships don't last long, as she also seems predisposed to finding fault with everyone over time. Our son's friends who have socialised with them on rare occasions report she has frequently ranted and raved at our son in public over several matters, including not being able to find solutions for her missing arm and damaged leg. The red flags surrounding us are hard to ignore.

My research of Khmer culture has included the suggestion that the women possess dollars for eyeballs and any man in a relationship with one will never be in full control of his own finances. I have heard criticisms from her about our son purchasing beer, yet she thinks nothing of buying designer gear and expensive cosmetics for herself. After they'd left I found a receipt from a jewellers for a ring costing over a thousand pounds which I later discovered she used to pay a fine for a traffic offence in Cambodia. It seems her obsession with money and material goods excludes any noticeable moral conscience.

Their plan is to return to England in November with her child, but as every plan they've made so far has not seen fruition I'm not holding my breath. Part of me wonders if they'll ever return. Either way, I have to prepare myself for more changes and talk myself into believing I can accept their decision if they choose to stay in Asia instead. The alternative option will mean the addition of a stranger's child into our family and this is a difficult one for me. I've never been the mother earth type or swooned around infants. After years of teaching, helping to raise a stepdaughter and already having twin step grandsons with no blood ties, I feel I've had enough. I'm ashamed my heart probably isn't big enough to take on a foreign baby with no links to our family.

At the same time I feel concerned about the child. After spending her first year of life in Cambodia and living most of it with relatives, how is she going to react to these almost virtual strangers whisking her away and flying thousands of miles to a cold and totally different culture? Although still very young, I envisage she'll feel very upset and frightened by all the changes and unfamiliar faces. I'm aware too my son has little or no experience of babies and has even declared previously he never wants children. With a disabled wife, he'll have more than his fair share of duties with the child, yet I'm not convinced he'll even recognise which end screams and which poops. I have voiced my suspicions that he will ultimately become stressed out with a house full of kids, though he has adamantly assured me there'll be no more, as his wife already regrets the one she has. Hardly a reassuring statement. And what of the real father? We know little about him but are aware he lives in England, so another niggle adds to the growing list.

We keep in touch for the next three months they spend in Cambodia, where things aren't as ideal as they seemed from our son's first visit. It's now the rainy season there and they've had to secure inferior accommodation to save funds. It's not long before our son ends up in hospital with food poisoning and is very distressed after a young girl in the next bed dies during the night. One of many motor cycle victims in a country with little legislation as regards health and safety. On the rare occasions we speak on the phone he claims everything is fine but I'm not convinced or reassured. Maybe it's my over active imagination, but I detect something in his voice, just as I had in his eyes when they'd stayed with us.

As their return to England draws closer they discover the child will need her own visa, causing more expense and delay. I'm quite concerned when I learn his wife has entered our son's name on the child's birth certificate, which is one of several necessary documents to secure the visa. The implications of such an action don't seem to bother her and I can't help pondering if lies and deceit come easily to her and what other things she's not been honest about.

As autumn days come to an end, we find ourselves travelling yet again to Heathrow to pick up the little family. In their absence we've secured and helped furnish a rented home for them about eight miles from where we live. We certainly couldn't entertain them living with us again and it only seems right they should have somewhere of their own to give them a chance to make a fresh start. This time his wife will have a visa for two years, so it's important to help them settle, particularly as winter is on the horizon and we have no idea how she will adjust to the season.

The plane lands on time and it's a comfort to see our son walking into the arrivals lounge after a long and worrying absence. As I hug him I turn to see his wife in a wheelchair escorted by a staff member and can't fail to notice the tears rolling down her face. I don't know the reasons for them, but suspect they are as many and complex as she seems to be. I walk over to hug her too, then bend to say hello to the little stranger on her knee. I think of this now as a defining moment in this bizarre story.

As we head for the car park, I can't help noticing how easy and caring my son is with the child he carries in his arms. He's caused a lot of problems and made some foolish mistakes, but at this moment I feel quite proud of him as I recognise what a big heart he has to take all this on and his obvious potential to be a loving and patient father.

The next few weeks are spent helping set up the new home and making adjustments for us all. Our son, a qualified criminologist, acquires a prestigious position and the welcome, steady income should mean more security. His wife is quite shocked to discover how cold it is and is amazed at the fact the summer trees now wear no leaves. With her disabilities, it will be difficult for her to find suitable clothing or footwear for severe weather, but as her walking ability is so limited she won't be travelling far without family transport, so it shouldn't be a major concern .

Being alone at home with the baby is her biggest tribulation. It's difficult for any young mother, but with her added problems and foreign background, it proves at times to make her resentful, lonely and unable to understand the nuclear families of England. My husband and I are still caring for three demanding and fragile parents and can only devote so much time to our son's situation and besides, harsh as it may sound, it was her choice to marry and come to live here.

However, the biggest surprise is the child and our reaction to her. She quickly finds a place in our hearts we'd never have imagined could have existed. Not only is she a cute little poppet in appearance, her nature proves to be calm and loving and her intelligence exceptional, despite the fact she has no language yet. A bond is very swift to form and she soon looks forward to seeing us, always smiling broadly and enjoying new experiences.

So, life ticks along for a while with some problems, some upsetting spats, some welcome family bonding and pleasant days. Christmas this year is far superior to the last, with a small child in our midst and the family able to all sit down at the table together with some peace and harmony restored.

But, come the New Year, my suspicions of what I've already predicted are confirmed. Another child will be added to the family and although this will be my first blood related grandchild, I can't help contemplating the complex difficulties should their relationship fail or they decide they can't hack life in England.

The baby is due on the auspicious date of September the 11th, but little do we know of the events life will throw at us before then.

River Of Tears

July 2008

When others talk of odd couples they usually have people they know in mind, but to me there's no odder couple than my own parents. I often think they originated from different planets rather than mere continents. From my first memories while living with our grandparents I can only recall them as very separate beings leading almost totally different lives. There were family holidays and outings, days spent with relatives and friends, but on the whole they spent their time apart, pursuing their own interests and mixing with their own companions. Being together often created a tense atmosphere or caused conflict, mostly instigated by our Mum, who is definitely the dominant one in their strange relationship and a bit of an excitement seeker; a social butterfly still searching for the man to match up to her own father, despite having a husband and children. Our Dad is a quiet, reserved man who probably prefers plants to people. My sister and I often contemplate whether we are adopted, as we can't imagine how they came together to make us, and if they did we suspect it may only have been twice. I guess we got used to things over the years, but we're pretty sure both moulds were broken when they made our parents. They both have some admirable qualities, haven't been bad parents and love us in their own way, though they've never been overly tactile or generous with praise. And of course, we love them both despite being aware their relationship has been nothing like those of many other parents.

Since they retired and eventually moved to the area where I live with my family, their habit of living separate lives has thrown up some problems. As their age increases and their health deteriorates the duty of care tends to fall on my shoulders more and more. Doctor's appointments have to be made and accompanied by me, as the idea of actually going anywhere together at this stage would probably cause panic attacks. Any stays in hospital require me to visit the one in a ward bed and the other left alone at home, as the notion of visiting each other would probably never enter their heads. I have power of attorney for both and my responsibilities continually increase as my mother's mental abilities deteriorate and my father develops more health problems requiring hospitalisation. I frequently write comical accounts of life in La La land as I call it, but in truth the decline in their ability to cope, the responsibilities of dealing with all their affairs and the heartache of watching them fade into shadows of the people they have once been is reaching crisis point. All this on top of our son's worrying situation starts to take its toll and there is little time to spare for our own activities, outings and holidays.

By the time our daughter-in-law has her first scan I guess we've accepted the fact there will be another child in the family. There are concerns of course. All I can envision is a family with financial, cultural, physical and emotional problems sinking further into the mire. Our son is working full time and long hours, returning home to tackle housework and caring for someone else's child. He already admits to feeling tired and stressed, so how will he cope with a newborn as well? Being disabled, how will his wife manage with a new baby and a toddler around the place? How will she feel being at home alone with two children and how will her little girl react to another child, being short of two herself and still adjusting to life in England? What will happen if the whole relationship goes belly up and a blood child is involved? But I'm sure most of us have been in a situation where possible scenarios threaten to swallow us up and have to come to the conclusion there's little we can do about any of it. After all, a new baby shouldn't be bad news, but rather something to rejoice in. Even my Mum, despite her understanding and memory rapidly deteriorating, works out she will have a first great-grandchild and seems quite thrilled by the idea.

In early spring, my husband and I leave for a much needed week's break in Majorca. While there we receive the news the baby will be a boy, swiftly followed by a worrying phone call from my sister, informing us my Mum has been admitted to hospital, with undiagnosed problems. Not really conducive to a relaxing holiday but thankfully by the time we return she's back home, though not in a very good state of health. The hospital has picked up on her dementia, but it seems there's little they can do. The same applies to the niggling health concerns no one seems able to identify. By the beginning of May she's back in a local hospital for assessment, very confused, frightened and longing just to return to the safety net of her own home.

During this phase our son and family move house, so as to be nearer his work and to have more room for the forthcoming addition. I silently shed tears as I scrub floors and surfaces at the house they are leaving, help shift heavy furniture into the new place, all the time worrying about my mother in hospital, scared and in denial of her deteriorating mental state. I've borne the brunt of her anger and frustration, knowing only too well these are symptoms of this heartbreaking condition but also acutely aware there is nothing I can do to change it.

The family settle into their new home, our little girl comes on in leaps and bounds, Mum comes home and eventually, after a long struggle I manage to secure some outside carers to help look after her. The relief is very welcome and on the strength of things looking brighter, in early summer we take our son and his family away for a week of glorious sunshine on the Isle of Wight. There are a few sticky moments and his wife being quite heavily pregnant by now needs a lot of help and rest. But it's a pleasure to watch her daughter enjoy her first visit to the seaside and I think we all feel a little more refreshed on return. It isn't to last.

I visit my parents the Friday afternoon after our return and meet Mum's lovely carer for the first time, witness Mum cleaner, more lucid and chatty than in a long time and as I leave their house later that afternoon, I offer up my private prayer of thanks.

The next morning, a grey and drizzly one, my husband and I spend a couple of hours at the gym about eight miles away. After I've showered and dressed, I come out to the car park to discover our car isn't there. I feel niggled that he doesn't think to tell me before driving off, but conclude hubby has nipped into town to do a bit of shopping, so I walk to the top of the nearby hill to wait for him. After a few more minutes I'm getting cold and agitated, so take out my mobile phone to call him. Unusually, there are five missed calls on it, two from my parent's, one from my son and two from a number I don't recognise. Instinctively, I know something is wrong.

I phone the unrecognised number first, which turns out to be a paramedic. I'm not sitting down as requested when he informs me my Mum has passed away and asks me to get to the house as swiftly as possible. I try to phone my husband but there appears to be no signal to his phone. Alone, in shock and not knowing what to do, I phone my son, knowing how much the news of his Nanna's death will upset him. He's gutted and sympathetic but says he's been trying to get hold of us to tell us his wife has lost all the water around the baby and has been rushed to hospital. I still can't contact my husband so have to stand waiting in torture until he arrives back, completely unaware of all that has happened.

The next few weeks pass in a blur of tears, grieving, formalities, the funeral I've dreaded all my life, while trying to support a frail father and offer support to my son and family. Son's wife is discharged but has to visit the hospital daily in order to check out the baby's condition. The plan is to help her pregnancy through to thirty-five weeks when it will be safe to deliver the baby by caesarean section. Every day carries a risk as we pray and wait with bated breath for what we now consider our treasured grandson.

Our prayers are answered on this occasion. My first official grandchild arrives in the world five weeks early, the day after my own birthday and just over three weeks from my Mum's passing. The river of tears threatens to reach bursting point as I welcome our new family member, contemplate the cycle of life, the fact my precious Mum didn't make it to see her great-grandchild, the acute awareness I am now in the position my Mum had been when I gave birth to my son and the concerns for the precarious future of us all. But life goes on doing what it will whether we like it or not and after loss, we cling with both hands to the hope new beginnings will transpire, hanging on by the thinnest of threads.

Take Me Home

February 2009

We all know change is one of life's certainties. Sometimes for the better, other times for worse and often just a heavy cloud of mystery suspended over the future. After the sudden death of my mother and the birth of my first blood grandchild I know life will never be the same and try to avoid contemplating the implications of these changes. Not being a natural optimist and having experienced some harsh blows I'm not about to start predicting an untroubled path ahead, but it has become obvious far too soon my days of caring and anxiety are far from over.

Even before my mother's funeral, we have to call out doctors and ambulances to my now eighty-eight-year-old father after minor falls and imagined heart attacks. I have always dreaded the day when there is only one parent left to care for and predicted correctly it would be my Dad, despite him being the older one. I know in some ways it's a blessing my Mum doesn't have to suffer any more of the indignity and frustration of dementia and admittedly in some ways it's a relief, even if a painful one for me, not to have to deal with the heartache of it on a daily basis. But I've loved my Mum for fifty-seven years of my life and have never spent more than a fortnight away from her, so the raw pain of loss is impossible to ignore and adjusting to life without her extremely difficult. I love my Dad too but have never had that close relationship some daughters have with their fathers, so feel my care is more of a duty than a loving role, which adds to my guilt. It creases me seeing him sitting in what had been my Mum's chair and I can never visit the house without battling tears, while putting on a brave face for the sake of my Dad. Losing a parent is one of life's hardest knocks and there's never a right time for it. If it happens early in life it seems cruel and people are left feeling deprived and resentful. Losing one late breaks your heart when you witness the deterioration and see the one left behind, old, lost and alone. Catch 22.

After a few weeks my father is admitted to hospital as a result of a bad fall and my own heartache is left dwindling in the background as I divide my time between his now empty home and visiting times at the hospital. Despite organising a personal alarm and attempting to secure some help with social services it's obvious he's not going to cope well alone, yet stubbornness and pride prevent him from admitting it.

My daughter-in-law has been awarded some paid help in the home due to her disabilities and having two young children, but this does not mean we are able to enjoy less input or feel things are settled with our son and family. I try to believe things might just work out and there are occasions I feel proud of my son for taking all this on and doing his best to prove they can cope, but at other times when his wife posts damning complaints on the internet and shows little gratitude to anyone trying to help, hope dissipates like morning mist and despair quickly replaces any positivity. Many times she announces she wishes she'd never come to "Bloody England," to use her own words and wants to go for a lethal injection as she feels so miserable. It upsets me as I'm sure there's far more to her problems than just her life here, and the scars run deep. It's almost impossible to imagine how the damage caused by trauma has affected her personality. How difficult it must have been surviving as a disabled female in a harsh and underprivileged country. It breaks my heart to think how much she has suffered in her short life and how the potential to be a beautiful soul has been tainted, but I'm far from perfect myself and cannot always overlook her problematic mood swings. It's pretty apparent she's lonely and struggling at home with two small children, but her own efforts to make any changes or improvements are sadly lacking. Although she obviously cares for her children and sees to their basic needs, her mothering skills leave a lot to be desired. There are occasions when we fear for the welfare of the children left alone in her care but are not in a position to voice our concerns too loudly. The helpers employed to assist her come and go as problems arise or they clash with her forceful personality, just as the friends she has sought out from all over the country are soon cast aside when they offend or disagree with her.

As a new year dawns so arrives the first trauma. We know our daughter-in-law can be over demanding, volatile and a drama queen and have learned not to react to her histrionic outbursts, as this tends to make matters worse. Her theatrical moods generally dissipate fairly quickly if she's just left to simmer. However, when she reports both her parents are unwell and her mother now in hospital with full blown AIDS and little hope of survival we are forced into a new and difficult situation. In her usual melodramatic way she insists she needs to return to Cambodia, with or without the children, and expects her trip to be financed. Always the cynical one, I'm not proud of the fact I inwardly question if there are ulterior motives behind her claims and if she's just looking for a way to visit Cambodia. And if she goes, there's always the question of whether she'll return. The marriage has lasted two years but still hasn't convinced me it's stable or sincere. Most of the time I witness a besotted, soft hearted young man trying to create a fairy tale world for his disabled wife, who appears to have unrealistic expectations. Admittedly she has suffered a great deal of trauma in life having lost her right arm after an accident, then suffering polio which has left her barely able to walk, but too often she seems to expect to be treated like a princess and frequently reacts like the one with a pea under her pillow.

Eventually, family discussion ensues and our daughter-in-law persuades us to believe her mother will not survive much longer, so she needs to see her for what could be the last time and allow her mother to meet her new grandson. My husband agrees to a loan to pay for her trip and it's decided the children will travel with her. Fears of how she'll cope and for the health and safety of the children have to be pushed aside as plans are hurriedly put in place. A flight is booked, necessary vaccinations carried out and passports sorted. Except they don't take into consideration the new baby cannot be added to his mother's passport, as being a British citizen he will need one of his own. This leads to a delay and results in our son's wife flying out to Cambodia with her daughter, leaving us to care for the baby at home while our son works. The following week, after securing a passport for the baby, he flies out with their son to join her for a few days, then returns alone to resume his work.

Three weeks later we await the return of our daughter-in-law and grandchildren to England. It's a tense and fraught time as we ponder how or even if, she'll manage the long journey back with two small children. Her flight will involve a stop at Hong Kong airport, where she should be greeted by a helper with a wheelchair, enabling her to transfer to the plane back to England. It's from there we receive a frantic phone call from her. The help hasn't arrived, both children are distressed and she has no idea what to do, ending her call with the statement she's returning to Cambodia. My husband springs into action, phones Hong Kong airport, who then manage to locate her and make sure she boards the flight to England.

It's a relief when the family are reunited and we can hopefully resume some semblance of normality as we know it. Our daughter-in-law complains loudly about planes, airports, staff, costs, weather and corruption but little is revealed about the state of her mother's health and her parents continue to thrive. Maybe it's been a case of amateur dramatics to secure a visit to Cambodia, but we feel we could not stand in her way. We are sure there will be more of these incidents in the future, but for the moment we are just thankful to have the family safely back on English soil.

My Dad continues to live like a deaf hermit in his own bubble and his main topic of conversation centres around the fact he'll turn ninety on his next birthday. He contemplates whether he'll reach it and informs me if he does, and can't look after himself, he doesn't want to. I remind him I don't possess a firearm but refrain from expressing the fact all his shopping, appointments, housework, laundry and problems are already dealt with by his daughter, so he isn't exactly living independently. His falls and call outs after pressing his lifeline continue to increase, which does nothing for my already frayed nerves. While my husband and I are away on holiday in Zante he has to be rescued from the bathroom in the early hours of the morning, where he's fallen and is trapped behind the door, involving the fire service as well as an ambulance. A fraught and exasperating three weeks in hospital ensue; professionals constantly relaying conflicting information and doing very little to address the problem of what to do about his increasing propensity to falls. Apart from moving him around wards, bagging up his laundry along with alien garments of other patients, keeping various charts of his blood pressure, pulse, temperature and bowel movements, we see very little evidence of any action. Ultimately, we decide to turn one of the downstairs rooms at his home into a bedroom in an attempt to limit the falls.

I spend a whole weekend alone attempting to create a bedroom from what was once a dining room where family visited, laughed, loved and shared stories. I walk into an empty house which has my mother's stamp on it everywhere. I move my Dad's bedding, clothing, medication and go about the business of clearing out drawers and cupboards full of memories from the past. It breaks my heart, yet even though my mind is screaming with the pain of it all I seem to have lost the ability to cry or grieve properly. I don't have time to analyse my own state of mind and maybe the warning signs are already apparent that I am functioning on autopilot and rapidly reaching saturation point.

My Dad returns home without any of the input promised from social services and despite living on one level, the falls continue. Being obstinate and a loner he refuses to join us for Christmas Day and it is no big surprise when the lifeline company phone just as I am about to dish up dinner for my own family.

So as one year ends and another begins, the familiar routine of ambulances, hospitals, attempting to secure help and failing continues. If only someone would listen.

Nothing Comes Easy

January 2010

I hadn't anticipated hospital visits at the start of a new year, but should hardly be surprised after so many similar scenarios. The usual lack of communication, contradictions, errors and broken promises is hardly surprising either, matters only made worse by some very severe winter weather. Hospital trips have become a familiar part of my life and my biggest fear is once all the visiting stops, I will be the next in line as a patient. But no good going down that imponderable road; one day at a time has to be my mantra.

I honestly believe Dad feels he's had enough of life and simply cannot be bothered with things any longer, but what are we to do? On occasion he reluctantly confesses he feels the time has come to accept some help and maybe move to wardened accommodation. However, we are never allowed to be present when professionals discuss things with him and it seems they are quite content to close the book after conversations with a ninety-year-old man who probably mishears or misunderstands everything they ask. Dad is severely deaf; the expensive hearing aid I'd spent hours organising for him just an ornament gathering dust on his mantelpiece, as he claims all it does is amplify sound.

I receive only phone calls from Social Services informing me Dad has refused any form of help and so the case is closed, then a second call from the ward notifying me they are about to discharge him. I ask the hospital if we need to fetch him, but they assure me transport is arranged and it would cause too many problems to cancel it. It occurs to me that Dad doesn't actually have any day clothes at the hospital, but no one has bothered to ask about that. Neither have they showed any concern about depositing him back at home in the middle of winter without ensuring the house will be heated and there is food in the fridge. Sadly, emptying beds in overstretched hospitals has become a common practice and more important than the practicalities of discharging elderly patients.

We wait for hours before an ambulance arrives. On one of the coldest nights of the year Dad is wheeled to the door wearing only short-sleeved cotton pyjamas, slippers and a small, flimsy blanket haphazardly draped over his shoulders. Two paramedics ask us if he is capable of walking inside.

'Yes,' we reply, 'but he needs his walking stick.'

'Where is his walking stick?' they ask.

'At the hospital the last we saw it.'

So, we've a ninety-year old man in hospital due to falls and they send him home without his walking stick? Finally, we settle Dad in his warm bed and leave with jangled nerves and rumbling stomachs.

The next day we go to check on him and unpack his belongings. There's a letter from the hospital for Dad's doctor which informs us the reason he's been in hospital is due to pneumonia. Well, who knew? Do they just make it up as they go along? The promises of Social Service input, home assessment, specialist stockings to aid circulation, daily visits from a community nurse and close assessment of his health have, as usual, come to nothing. We also have to drive in hazardous conditions to the hospital to retrieve his walking stick. No apologies, no staff available to talk to, no notes left on the ward and I predict, no chance of anything changing in the future.

At this stage my sister and I decide to compose a letter of complaint. We express our concerns about his safety, living alone and the fact no one in authority will listen to us when we voice our opinion he needs supervision and a lot of outside help. We are not particularly optimistic it will achieve anything, but mounting frustration and fear are becoming too much to live with.

Another bump in the rocky road of life arrives when we receive a phone call from our son to say he's received a letter informing him his wife's visa is about to expire and her application for indefinite leave has been declined by the Home Office. Their reasons? Apparently, she has failed to attend classes and take a test about English heritage. The test, inaptly named "Life in the U.K," is a ridiculous, multiple-choice paper composed of questions which I doubt any U.K citizen would be able to answer correctly. The original invitation to take the test was accompanied by a letter, explaining if she was unable to attend due to disability or other reasons, she should send a doctor's note and that would suffice. She cannot walk far, doesn't drive and has two small children. They acquired the requested note, sent it off and expected that would be that. Our son could have taken her I suppose, but he has work commitments and is not of the opinion a test asking who was on the throne in 1465 or what percentage of the population is Jewish of much relevance. Classes in English and Maths would be more useful, yet she was initially refused those on the grounds she needed to be a resident here for at least a year.

The Home Office insensitively stated they have looked into her application and compared her case to others, concluding she has less right to stay here. They suggest the family take up residence in Cambodia. They make no reference to the fact my son is English and has a responsible job which he could never match in a third world country. They claim her daughter did not arrive here until 2009, when in fact she's been in England since 2007, is happily settled in nursery school and having an English father, has a right to claim dual nationality. There is no mention of their son, born here and a British citizen by right. Three out of four in this family have English roots and the authorities think it best they bugger off to Asia? Over my dead body.

Add to this the fact our son's family live here, we are the only grandparents the children have ever known, they are law-abiding citizens who make no claims from the state and are doing their best to improve the quality of their lives through hard, honest work and it is grossly unfair.

Of course, they will appeal against this decision and hopefully win, but we could do without the hassle in our already stressful and complex lives. I can't think beyond that; if the situation arose where the family had to move to Cambodia I think that would be the final straw and I'd just want to fade away. There's only so much fight we can contend with and I'm rapidly approaching overload.

Our own letters of appeal are swiftly sent out and the story hits the local newspapers. As a result, the regional television news company contact them and request an interview. It's really strange watching my son and his little family on the television. It makes me feel proud of them all. How can anyone think it fair to take a disabled mother away from her children or deprive two tinies of the only life they've ever known here? Eventually the Home Office agree to fully review her application and admit mistakes have been made. The letter they send is full of grammatical and spelling errors and it's tempting to suggest whoever composed it should be made to take the required test themselves.

She is eventually granted a three year, indefinite stay in the U.K, a bit of a contradiction in terms. She will have to study and learn the correct responses to the Life in the U.K test and pass it before she is allowed to apply for British citizenship. When, or if she succeeds she'll be able to acquire a passport. Her Cambodian passport has expired so she cannot travel, and the Cambodian Embassy in England refuse to renew it, claiming she needs to do that in Cambodia. A typical example of how the corrupt, bizarre Cambodian culture operates.

Although I"m relieved and obviously want the family to remain on our shores, our daughter-in-law is proving to be more demanding, volatile and resentful. I'm ashamed to admit there are times when I could lash out at her myself and I also notice our son becoming more tense, short tempered and exhausted with it all. When she posts damning comments about her life and family in England on social media for all to see, I'll confess it makes me livid, but any criticism is greeted with stony silence or hysterics, as if she's the one who has been wronged.

When we've looked after the children all weekend so they can have a break away, then she sneaks off for a nap on return, my patience is stretched to the limits, but a wry comment means all hell breaks out once the princess is aware she's been criticised.

When she expects loans running into thousands to pay for her parent's hospital fees, then flies off the handle and sulks for a week when we tell her we don't have access to such funds, we see no hope for a settled future. I'm pretty sure she's sending money to her family back in Cambodia, as is their custom, and I'm also aware of how many designer products she seems to acquire. Fair enough if you have the money to spare, but they don't, and even though I try to diplomatically point out we are not a private child minding and banking service, nothing changes.

But then other times, when laughter prevails and we see the strong, individual and determined side of her character, a glimmer of hope that things just might work out flickers. When we witness the enquiring looks of strangers wondering about our family and how it all came about, then it often gives us a sense of pride in being unusual. For now all I can ask for is some time free of hassle and trauma, in order to maybe eventually enjoy some peace of mind but my hope it will one day happen proves to be short lived.

Sick And Tired

May 2010

I learned a lot at Grammar School, mainly about snobbery, injustice, victimisation, pressure and fear. I left at eighteen with more complexes than exam passes, several bad habits, a case full of Beatles memorabilia, some good friends plus a few enemies after I'd pulled and hung on to the best looking boy in the school. That relationship lasted on and off for ten years, whereas the friendships either ended after the last day of school or drifted slowly into the past as life and circumstances altered.

Yet again, it is thanks to technology many of those friendships have been rekindled, blossomed and some new ones added. In the early days of the internet, before social media sadly took over, it seemed almost miraculous that we were given the opportunity to link up with old school friends and people from the past. Reunions have become part of life now. I remember the first one I attended, feeling nervous and not knowing what to expect. After getting over the shock of entering a room full of elderly people, then realising I must look like one as well, it was a wonderful experience to reconnect with friends from the past. I always enjoy them despite my husband's initial jealousy and disapproval. Things have improved to some extent once he meets people and realises they are mere human beings and not a threat.

It's on a Saturday when I'm looking forward to one of these reunions in the evening that I visit my Dad's house and discover he has fallen yet again and is trapped behind the entrance door to his lounge. I have to fetch a neighbour to help me move him enough to enter and it's obvious I need to call for an ambulance. The plug on his alarm is out of its socket, so pressing his panic button has failed to contact anyone and he has obviously been on the floor all night and is in very poor shape. An ambulance eventually arrives and the hospital later inform us he's broken a hip bone and it seems likely his general health is not good enough for him to withstand surgery. What happens now I just don't know, but whatever the outcome it's likely to be a very long haul with a lot of care, changes and paperwork ahead. I cannot back out of the reunion as I'm the organiser and there is little can be done anyway. Needless to say, I don't enjoy it as much as anticipated and ponder if there'll ever be a time when a carefree outing is possible.

A few days later a consultant calls to inform us that all things considered the risk of an operation has to be taken, as otherwise there is no way to relieve pain. Obviously considering Dad's age and frail condition the concern over his recovery is very high.

The afternoon of the operation I'm a gibbering wreck and can't describe all the feelings, thoughts and scenarios that occupy my thoughts. Nothing is straightforward when considering the future for someone of his great age, but he survives and is quite lucid the following day, though obviously exhausted, needing rest and the expert care of hospital staff. He looks like he's gone ten rounds in the boxing ring and is very, very frail. The nurses ask if I can persuade him to take in some fluid as he's not eating or drinking too well. He complains he'd be happier sipping lager than orange juice, so there's still a glimmer of his old self in there and I assure him I'll be drinking his share later. It's going to be a long, hard road before we can breathe easily or consider what happens next.

In the following days we're told Dad has to make more effort with eating, drinking and movement if his recovery is going to take place. He's rather lazy, but at his age he has a right to be. He doesn't seem concerned or as if he can be bothered with much and I quite understand but feel helpless as to what to do. Life doesn't come with a get out clause and none of us know what lies ahead. I have a feeling whatever it is, it's not going to be very pleasant, but I have my very negative head on right now.

We're looking at weeks more of hospitalisation, physiotherapy and trying to get some input from the powers that be to help us come to some conclusions. I'm feeling much like Dad, with little energy or enthusiasm for anything. Although I should be used to these sort of situations by now, for some reason this latest episode has knocked out all my stuffing. I'm just feeling so weary of everything and struggling to cope with each day.

I can't remember the last time I fell asleep feeling relaxed, had a dreamless night or woke up feeling refreshed. Insomnia, nightmares and morning apathy have become a way of life I can't seem to do much about. I know worry solves nothing and am aware everyone goes through bad phases, but I honestly feel exhausted with the longevity of anxieties I've endured. I try not to feel sorry for myself but am so damned tired of everything, at the same time berating myself for feeling this way.

I'm tired of caring. I'm tired of coping single-handed with the problems of old age. I'm tired of never having a day without responsibility. I'm tired of dealing with the troubles of family members and trying to slap on a smile when I really want to scream. I'm tired of bad news, fighting in the face of adversity and failing to live up to expectations. I'm tired of my life and I'm tired of my own attitude. Even if I get away from it all for the odd day, it's still all there in my head.

I'm tired of hospitals. In the last five years I've had a parent in hospital seventeen times. There were many times before that, including the three years my husband was in and out of them after horrendous problems from a hip replacement. I used to be able to cope with it, but now I feel literally sick every time I go through the hospital doors.

Dad has good and bad days but seems very tired of it all too. Sometimes he'll perk up and the nurses joke with him. He's not a demanding patient, quiet and polite and nurses always take to him. In fact, one said she wanted to marry him the other day. I told her I wished she would and that would ease my situation. They have him sussed. They commented on his poor hearing but are aware he'd hear if someone announced there was a ten pound note on the floor. They realise he'd be far more willing to take in fluid if it contained alcohol. But pleasantries and light-hearted jokes won't solve any problems. I'm fully aware that a broken hip in someone his age is a serious problem and often the start of other major conditions. The operation has been deemed a success, but he's still not walking and other minor symptoms need treating before any decisions can be made. No one mentions where we're going from here and his future care plays on my mind only I suspect. I do not want to place him in a care home against his will, but neither can I cope with the nightmare of continuous falls at home.

Eventually, my sister and I are invited to a formal complaints meeting as a result of the letter we'd sent before this latest fall, but as suspected our concerns are dismissed, and it's obvious all members around the table have closed ranks and are unwilling to accept our insistence Dad can no longer cope alone at home.

After ten weeks the hospital inform us Dad is adamant about returning home and as he is of sound mind, no one has the power to make him do otherwise. We point out he's said otherwise to us and being profoundly deaf probably hasn't understood the conversations at the hospital. We feel strongly had we been allowed to be with him during discussions things would have been different, but the hospital still constantly refuse our presence. We are assured a very intensive care package will be put in place to assist him at home.

It's all systems go to reorganise his home yet again, put appropriate aids in place and fill his fridge. My sister and I go to visit him in hospital for what we think will be the last time, only to discover the doors to his ward are locked due to an outbreak of a norovirus, and no one is allowed in or out until the ward has been free of the virus for seventy-two hours. I guess it's too much to expect anyone to have informed us before we set out. The care package we've set up is lost.

Problems abound and Dad's discharge from hospital is delayed twice more, when blood tests reveal some abnormality that needs investigation, followed by a second outbreak of norovirus on the ward, but finally, after three months, he arrives home and despite carer's visiting four times a day there is only so much they can do and it isn't easy to cast aside concerns of when the next call out will be.

It has taken many falls and hospital admissions to secure any help for Dad, but despite four visits a day from care assistants, the falls continue day and night, some resulting in hospital visits, some less serious. Without twenty-four hour supervision there is always the fear of hazardous falls occurring. I have reached the point where every telephone call brings on a feeling of dread, along with fighting a constant battle to ward off depression and anxiety attacks. I can't help blaming myself to some extent as I'm perfectly aware others deal with far worse situations, and I reproach myself for my faults, my failures, my weaknesses, that ensure I don't cope as well as others. I should be able to handle my dark feelings, but there is something in me I can't control that makes me feel inferior, inadequate, a failure. I know I ought to look at things differently with strength and hope, but I can't, and find it difficult to forgive myself for that. I try to push my mounting sense of dread to one side. I tell myself I have to keep going and everything will work out, but there is always that inner voice convincing me it won't.

Slipping Away

February 2011

We're helping our son and family move house again, shifting furniture, scrubbing surfaces, emptying boxes, hanging curtains and entertaining two lively toddlers. Problems with the family are frequent and obvious; another move more a potential hazard than a reason to celebrate. I suspect my son's rose-coloured spectacles are slipping, and sadly I'm never sure either he or his wife are completely honest or trustworthy. In the midst of the house move we receive an early morning call from one of Dad's carers to say he's fallen and an ambulance is on its way. Thankfully he is not taken to hospital, but in a rare, emotional conversation, he confesses maybe the time has come to consider a care home. Knowing this is the last thing he wants but realising we cannot carry on this way it breaks my heart to see him almost in tears. As a last resort we decide to move his bed into the lounge so he will be virtually living in one room, but we both know this is the end of the line.

Call outs continue and one afternoon, returning from his home because he needed help to get out of his chair I wonder where on earth this is all heading. I will find out much sooner than expected. My own health has not been very good and I seem to catch every minor bug going, but circumstances leave little time to rest or recuperate.

The following morning I'm blasted from sleep by the telephone. It's the lifeline company who inform me Dad has pressed his alarm again, but they cannot hear him speaking. Annoyed at yet another call out and having only just woken up I tell them I can't get to his house right away as my husband is out golfing and I'm not ready. I ask what they expect me to do about it and receive the curt reply, 'Well, he is your father.' Thankfully, a friend close by is at home and offers to drive me to the house when I call her. Thank goodness she does.

We arrive to find the street is cordoned off and several emergency vehicles are parked in various locations. I discover Dad in a wheelchair about to be taken to hospital and it's obvious he's in a very poor state and the house has been subject to a fire. The shock hits me hard, but there's no time to dwell on it.

It's later confirmed Dad had fallen yet again, but this time managed to tumble onto a halogen heater which then set fire to the curtains, which then fell onto his television and so on. It's purely by chance a passing paramedic who knows of my Dad's history decided to stop by, and it was only when he managed to open the side door, which thankfully was unlocked, the full extent of the situation became apparent. He literally dragged Dad from the building and thanks to his efficiency alone had alerted the necessary emergency services. It's a miracle Dad survived and a further miracle I wasn't the one to open the door to the house or I may have gone up with it. I'm furious about how things were handled by the lifeline company and the years I've wasted telling everyone involved that my father is not safe to live alone, yet had he died in the fire I would never have forgiven myself.

Dad has to be admitted to a hospital in the city with a specialist burns unit, as opposed to the usual local hospital. The difference is instantly apparent. All the staff are caring, efficient, organised and helpful. They involve me in discussions and ask opinions, which I've never been allowed before. They treat Dad with respect, dignity, humour and genuine concern. As a result, he is much more responsive than he's ever been in hospital before.

He's obviously frail and has severe injuries, but it's agreed by all we will now have to find a suitable care home as he cannot return to his house. It will need an awful lot of restoration before it's habitable. I cannot go inside it as it is under investigation and it would be too upsetting anyway. It's going to be another long haul as we deal with insurance companies, renovation, selling the house, finding a suitable care home and sorting out finances.

We are fortunate to find a place available in an excellent care home close by; a family run establishment with a small, devoted and stable staff. Dad settles in reasonably well, though he doesn't mix with other residents or make any effort to join in activities, which is what we would have anticipated. The main thing is he is now safer, with people on hand when there are falls or other health needs.

Problems and tensions with our son and his Cambodian princess of a wife continue. Patching things up becomes the norm, but their situation I know will always be unpredictable, unstable and we'll never know the whole truth. I frequently spend a long time on the phone listening to her concerns and complaints but conclude they are both to blame in some respects and still have a lot of growing up to do. This often makes me want to bang their heads together, but I refuse to entertain family warfare or contemplate how I'd feel if she decided to return to Cambodia with the children. Restraint is often difficult to maintain but a necessity when it's the only way to avoid conflict.

At this stage I am advised by my doctor to attend counselling sessions as it's becoming obvious I'm struggling. I do not want to take medication as it has been of little help in the past, and I can well live without the side effects. Counselling may help in some cases, but when you know the reasons why you're feeling low and anxious, there is little anyone can do to change that. I do come away with more letters after my name however, after being diagnosed with post traumatic stress disorder to add to the rest of my mental health conditions. But again, there is limited treatment or much help available.

While my husband's mother, at the age of ninety-seven survives a stay in hospital and continues to battle on in her own home, rarely asking for help, my Dad in the care home seems to have virtually given up. He needs further surgery on his burns, after which he spends most of his time in a horizontal position, rarely getting dressed or leaving his room. The falls continue and we are still involved in hospital visits, but at least the lifeline callouts in the middle of the night are a thing of the past.

The first fall at the care home which requires hospitalisation results in yet more frustration and anger. It's the first time I've seen my Dad extremely agitated in hospital. The nurses seem more concerned about his alcohol intake than caring for his physical and emotional needs, one of them even fetching an empty bottle of whisky to show me how many units of alcohol it contains. I point out to them my Dad has enjoyed a drink for most of his life, I've never seen him drunk, and at ninety-one it seems rather extreme to ask him to become tea total.

When the time comes for him to be discharged I receive a probing telephone call from the hospital asking if I know how he has acquired so many bruises, the reasons why he keeps falling, and how long he's lived in a care home, concluding the hospital will not be able to send him back there until they've carried out an assessment. I think it may be obvious I'm rather annoyed after informing the caller no one has ever bothered before and he's frequently been sent home to an empty house with no concerns about his injuries or safety. Suddenly, after years of fighting and attempting to convince them he is not fit to live alone, they've decided to intervene. It doesn't take a genius to work out they've had instructions to investigate, in case his injuries have been sustained by neglect or mistreatment in the care home. Nothing can be further from the truth and it makes my blood boil to think of all the neglect and indifference we've suffered in the past by professionals on countless occasions.

Thankfully Dad is back in the care home when I receive a call on the morning of Halloween to say they are concerned about his condition and will send for a doctor. By the time the doctor arrives he has slipped away peacefully. It's sad and upsetting of course, but we feel Dad had simply had enough. Despite all the accidents and trauma he's suffered over recent years there aren't many who can claim to have survived ninety-one years and then have the simple phrase "old age," recorded as the cause of death.

We wish Dad had made more of his life and taken advantage of the facilities in the care home, but that was his choice and his way. A quiet and private man right to the end.

Change is the only constant in life and as such I know the next year will bring more and hopefully better ones. It will be the first year I will have no parental responsibilities, which evokes a huge cauldron of mixed emotions for me. It will be strange and difficult to come to terms with. I've always dreaded the day I'd be an orphan. I'm not sure how I feel right now, but I'm struggling. Definitely pensive and sad of course, as well as battling with the bigger picture and pondering the future.

Sticky Situation

January 2012

Nine days into the New Year and I'm already feeling this is going to be another difficult one. It's five years to the day of my son's bizarre marriage, things have kicked off again, and I can't see a happy ever after on the horizon.

Our daughter-in-law has succeeded in becoming the centre of attention once again when she hysterically announces her father in Cambodia has been involved in a serious accident at work and is in hospital. In her usual drama queen manner she's predicting his demise and demanding to go out there, with no regard for the expense, her family here or the children's schooling. Admittedly, it's a long time since she last visited, but the timing makes me feel suspicious. It was only a short while after I'd lost my mother when she made the claims her own was at death's door and now, after only a few weeks without my Dad, her own is allegedly fighting for his life. I feel so guilty for even questioning her claims and even worse contemplating whether she does these things to compete on an emotional level. Lack of trust is chipping away at my determination to be a tolerant, empathetic, understanding person and I'm ashamed my dark mind can think such twisted thoughts. I would never voice them of course. Even a calm discussion as to why it's not practical for her to drop everything and fly to Cambodia results in theatrics.

As a result of not complying with her wishes we've all been wiped from her Facebook friends yet again, she's refused to join our son on an arranged night out to a party and has threatened to sell the iPhone I bought her for Christmas to finance her fare. I am also accused of not knowing my own son and always believing him over her. According to her, she's the victim, he gives her nothing and is cruel to her, she does everything for him and the world and his wife are responsible for all her problems, as she creates none. There may be some justification in her claims but she refuses to acknowledge that both people involved in situations, positive or negative, are responsible. I am not unsympathetic to her feelings or the fact she misses her family and her country, but she is proving over and over again that she has little consideration for anyone other than herself, is demanding, volatile, unreasonable and prone to causing confrontation, no matter how reasonable people try to be. My skills as a mediator are limited, and it's becoming a waste of time even trying to reason with her.

The difference now is I think my son's rose-coloured glasses have finally dropped off, and he's reaching the point where he's willing to admit he's made a big mistake and things cannot continue this way. Our son and the children stay with us the night of the party and I'm pleased he's decided to attend without her, despite things being so fraught between them. She claims she's staying at home, but again my lack of trust and her history of lying make me doubt that's true. The following evening, when he arrives back home with the children, she isn't in, he has no key, her phone is switched off and he is genuinely worried something may have happened to her. She finally arrives home at midnight and continues ranting. Not the actions of a caring mother or wife in my humble opinion.

I have no idea where we go from here. I do know he will have got up with the kids every morning as usual, washed, dressed and fed them before taking them to school, then taken time away from his demanding job to collect them after school, meaning he has to make up the time at work later. I imagine she'll have stayed in bed as usual, nursing her wounds and be on her phone and laptop complaining to anyone who will listen about her awful life and husband.

Later in the week we're informed her father has died of his injuries which makes me feel even more guilty, but I still believe her behaviour and some of the things she's said are totally out of order. She did not approach the subject of going to Cambodia in the correct way, but then, that is how she is. Surely she wouldn't lie about something so devastating?

Any doubts must be cast aside, as the situation is now a different one. We try to reassure her that even if she had left for Cambodia immediately, she would not have arrived there in time and there was little she could have done about it all anyway. We understand if she feels she needs to go back to support her family and attend any funeral rites and offer to pay for her flight as well as helping with the kids in her absence. However, when she asks to borrow two thousand pounds on top of that, we have to draw the line and decline.

Research leads me to believe the daughters in a Cambodian family are expected to pay for funerals, which seems rather bizarre and impractical, but I have always tried to respect her culture as best I can. There are four other daughters in her family, but they probably believe all westerners are filthy rich and can afford anything and everything. I'm also aware my daughter-in-law is not daft and realises I will have inherited a modest amount of money, but I do not like to think my Dad worked all his life to pay for a stranger's funeral. I know she would probably try to pay the money back, but that would make things difficult for them over a long period of time and I could not stand by and witness them struggling further, particularly as their relationship is shaky and may not last the course. I feel bad about it all, but am not prepared to cough up that amount of money in these circumstances.

I believe she is afraid her family in Cambodia will ask for money she hasn't got and I sympathise with her when she eventually decides going out there in sad circumstances would probably only make her feel worse, so she decides not to go. She refuses to discuss the situation with us. I also believe she is understandably depressed and would maybe benefit from medical intervention on that front, but she won't discuss that either.

When the family next visit us our son and the children seem fine but she is sullen, uncommunicative and disinterested. It's obvious she doesn't want to be here and though I realise she is bound to be very upset by her father's death, there is nothing we can do about it and she has two small children to care for here, where she has chosen to settle.

We again offer to pay for her to visit Cambodia if she feels it would help, but without further excessive funds she doesn't seem to want to go. She won't open up and discuss the matter or her feelings, and we suspect she's blaming our son and ourselves for her father's death, claiming if we'd supplied the money immediately for an operation it may have saved his life. I don't know all the facts, the customs, the truth or what happens next, but one thing I do know is I'm rapidly getting to the end of my rope with her very unfair, harsh and ungrateful attitude. I've been making allowances for five years now and I'm teetering on thin ice. I realise it's important to take cultural differences into consideration and from experience I know she will deal with things her own way and eventually come round, but I also know I am reaching breaking point.

I wish I was a coper, I wish I was strong, I wish I was tougher because some days life just seems too much to deal with. Why are we humans given so much feeling if it means hurting so much? I could cope with going through the motions if it wasn't for feelings. Why can't we switch them off and just do what we have to do each day without them? Where do they come from? Why can't we control them? Why do they threaten to swallow us up when all we're trying to do is just get by? Or maybe it's me. Maybe I'm lacking something which enables others to survive, maybe I've failed to work out how to carry on through sheer determination or maybe I'm just selfish. Unlike some, I have family and friends, but too often no-one considers I'm still grieving, still sorting out formalities after losing my Dad, still involved in the heartbreaking task of clearing his house and still feel invisible. Sometimes you can feel desperately lonely even when surrounded by friends and family.

Things will calm down I suspect, but if they return to any semblance of normality we are all aware it won't be long before there's another altercation and the cycle will continue and it just cannot go on. Our concerns, are of course, for the children and our son, though I do not wish any harm to her, but realise she's never going to change when she can't get her own way.

Even as an elderly orphan it seems the slings and arrows will continue flying in my direction and as I age I'm finding it more difficult to dodge them.

Living On A Prayer

December 2012

I took early retirement from teaching after it had become unbearable, thanks to a ruthless boss and an awful year of severe depression. My husband retired from his Headteacher's post at the same time which with hindsight was maybe not the best idea. However, despite our differences and difficult patches we hoped to enjoy a retirement without the pressures of a very demanding career and looked forward to a new phase in our lives. At this stage my parents and his widowed mother were fairly fit and our son still at university. We hoped to travel and almost bought a motorhome, but thought we'd wait until my husband had recovered from an imminent operation. A wise decision as it turned out.

My husband developed severe arthritis very early in life and will always need medication to help deal with it. The condition is partly a result of playing sport most of his life and suffering consequent injuries. He's been pretty stoic about it and continued to play cricket despite it probably being an unwise choice. Many a time spectators have grimaced as he's limped away from the crease. By the time we retired his left hip was proving very troublesome and the only answer would be a hip replacement, which he proceeded to schedule at a private hospital.

Several weeks after the operation it was discovered he'd developed an infection around the prosthesis which then had to be removed. We then had to wait a few months while he took antibiotics and without a hip bone in place he relied on crutches to get about. Not an ideal start to our retirement. A second hip replacement went ahead, but whatever the infection was, it failed to be eradicated, resulting in another removal of the hip joint and another six months relying on crutches while he was left with no hip. It was a very trying time during which he could do very little or get around much, though thankfully switching to an automatic car still enabled him to drive. Most duties were left for me to tackle and his constant presence along with the responsibilities took its toll. To this day I still hone in on the sound of crutches clacking from quite a distance away, and the familiar sound I've lived with over many long periods of time still makes me shudder.

Apart from diagnosing his condition as a Staphylococcus infection we received little information or explanation. Annoyed and worried, I researched his condition and the treatment he was receiving, in an effort to discover why he'd suffered two failed hip replacements. I discovered the antibiotic he was taking after the second failure was the only one to successfully treat MRSA, and yet the hospital adamantly denied its presence in his system. At that time private hospitals could not be held responsible for any ensuing problems after treatment, and I was virtually told to prove it if I didn't believe their claims that he'd just "drawn the short straw," to use their words.

It took almost two years before my husband was infection free and able to keep a prosthetic hip in place, though he was left with a gruesome scar, one leg slightly shorter than the other and an inability to walk without a bit of a John Wayne gait. The hospital advised him to always have a flu injection each year and a warning he may be more prone to infections than the average person.

Over the years he has had several strange and sometimes undiagnosed illnesses, as well as some severe arthritic attacks which leave him barely able to function. Thankfully, on the whole he is a strong and resilient man, so is generally able to live life as he wishes, though no doubt he'd prefer to still play sport rather than watch it on the television. I've noticed several times after he receives an injection or an insect bite he'll take ill and I ponder if whatever was in his system during the failed hip operations is the root cause. We've visited America several times during these years and on return he almost always develops some peculiar, debilitating symptoms and although tested for malaria, lyme disease and other rare conditions, they are never fully diagnosed.

Christmas is on the horizon once more when he complains one evening of a sore eye and on closer inspection it's noticeably red and swollen. The next morning the swelling is worse, his whole face becoming inflamed and his left eye almost fully closed. Fortunately, some friends who are visiting are able to take him to hospital as there is no way he can see to drive. He is sent home and given an appointment to return in the afternoon, by which time it's almost possible to witness the swelling expanding by the minute. Friends again drive him to the hospital and when I call him later in the evening he confirms he's being kept in on an antibiotic drip but doesn't seem overly concerned or in too much discomfort.

The following day I call his mobile, but it goes straight to answerphone. I call the hospital and am informed without any explanation my husband is no longer a patient but has been transferred to a hospital in the city. Mystified, I call that hospital and after a lot of delay and confusion I'm informed he's in an operating theatre and a surgeon will phone me later to explain. Anxious and unable to understand what is happening, the long wait seems interminable and when the call finally comes it is not in any way reassuring. Details are scanty, direct questions unanswered and all I am told for sure is that my husband is still in surgery and they will phone again when procedures are completed. I ask if he's in any danger and receive no reassuring response.

Alone and terrified, I feel the dreaded chemicals in my brain release and flow like a tidal wave as my mind attempts to take on board the possible outcome of this sudden and unexpected trauma. It's only four years since I lost my mother and I still miss her every day, just over a year since my father died, only a few short months after the horrendous fire which still haunts me on a regular basis. My mother-in-law at ninety-eight is deteriorating rapidly and has spent several spells in hospital. Things between my son and his problematic wife are continuing to go downhill and there has been frequent talk of divorce, the children being the only paper thin incentive keeping them together. Things deteriorated further when in the midst of their disputes and disharmony his wife had another meltdown after informing us her mother in Cambodia had died. Again I felt guilty for the niggle of doubt as to whether she was telling the truth or merely ensuring she was the centre of attention amongst distressing times. Surely it can't be true that now my husband is fighting for his life? Just how many times can your world fall apart?

I curl up in a foetal position pressed into the corner of the settee, the familiar sensations of chronic depression hovering and threatening to take over my already fragile state of mind. More of the hooks tenuously anchoring me to life for so long start to let go, and I can barely hold myself together. Eventually, I manage to call some friends who stay with me until I receive the next phone call. It's revealed my husband is seriously ill and will likely require further surgery. The exact diagnosis is not yet available, but specialists are pretty sure he has an extremely rare and serious form of a Streptococcus A infection, and he is now in intensive care in an induced coma, where he will remain for at least a week.

I have never been a big fan of Christmas but making a forty mile round trip daily to the hospital, often in inclement weather, while others rush around in a panic worrying about the weight of turkeys and what to buy for the family parrot only exacerbates the feeling. Spending Christmas Day sitting by the bedside of a comatose figure being kept alive by beeping machines, while observing other visitors wracked with anxiety and pain as they await news of seriously ill relatives, some of them children, makes you realise not everyone has reason to be feeling frivolous and jolly at this time of year. Something very few seem to take into consideration.

Over the next few days my stepdaughter, son and I keep a constant vigil at the hospital knowing only that he is being treated with the correct anti biotic, but machines are doing all the work to keep him alive. It's frightening when nurses frequently leave the room to fetch one of five specialists to check on their concerns and hard for us to understand the medical terms and strange symbols on the many machines. We know he'll be returning to the operating theatre to check there is no more infection, and if that is the case more aggressive surgery will be necessary. Without using the exact words we understand this infers the removal of the left eye, but nothing is more important than the assurance he will survive. Our relationship may be far from perfect, we have many times when disharmony dominates our daily lives, but no way do I feel could I face a life without him.

Keep Holding On

January 2013

Alone, like a storm-tossed wreck, I find it very difficult to concentrate on even basic tasks at home, as well as attempting to keep my own mental state stable enough to cope. Matters are made worse when my stepdaughter and husband's brother, an unsociable, confirmed bachelor still living with his ninety-eight-year old mother, decide between them it is best not to inform her that her eldest son is in hospital, fearing the shock might be too much for her. Fobbing her off with the lie he is just ill at home, they neglect to consider the fact it is me she phones every day to see how he is, and lying through my teeth, pretending he is resting in bed is something I bitterly resent and it does little to help me in any way.

After a long, agonising week, we are able to breathe more easily when it's confirmed the infection is under control and progress is being made, though there is still a long way to go. Streptococcus infections generally manifest themselves as a sore throat or a skin rash and are easily treated, but for whatever reason it had developed into the life threatening condition known as Necrotising Fasciitis in my husband's case. Inaccurately described as the flesh eating disease, it enters the skin through any abrasion or small cut and left untreated it would have killed him within forty-eight hours. It is more common for the bacteria to infect limbs, but as that generally results in amputation, in some ways my husband has been lucky, as the blood flow to the face is better. The five specialists assigned to his treatment have only seen a few cases in their combined eighty years experience.

He has to be slowly brought round from the induced coma and is obviously disturbingly agitated, requiring repeats of sedation at every attempt. There are brave faces in every direction, but until we know he will not be permanently disabled or damaged by all he's been through it's still a time of tremendous tension, anxiety hanging like a dark, impenetrable cloud each time we visit the hospital. Once conscious, he's moved to a high dependancy ward, though with a tracheotomy in place and still attached to several machines he is unable to speak, eat or drink. Not an easy situation for a man who likes to be in control of everything. Communication is difficult, but we are more confident he is going to be okay. He will face months of convalescence, skin grafts and reconstruction surgery, but taking one day at a time has become a necessity.

I sit at home alone on New Year's Eve, not making resolutions or celebrating but still feeling deeply disturbed. I've spent years caring for parents and dealing with the traumas of my son's bizarre family. Now I face a very uncertain future and the daunting task of caring for a very difficult patient. Yet again, I will start the new year with hospital visits and dare not even think what the next one might bring.

After several weeks in hospital, undergoing intensive treatment by specialists, my husband is finally allowed to come home. He looks very unwell. He's been given botox injections to keep his left eye closed, has dressings over the left side of his face and only sight in one eye at present. He has mounds of medication to take and is obviously frail and finding it difficult to get around the house. We have a winding staircase and only one toilet upstairs, so I'm very concerned for his safety and ability to manage daily essentials in such a poor state of health. Thankfully, the infection has been quashed and he will recover, albeit over a long period of time. But despite the relief, I have a feeling the trials we face now, as he recovers, are going to prove difficult. The familiar negative inner traits begin to rise, slowly and ominously like serpents from a deathly black lair, but I know this cannot be all about me, and must fight back.

Nurses visit daily to change the dressings and monitor his progress, and he will face many more hospital visits, including reconstruction of his face around the eye. We were promised information sheets and advice lists once he was discharged but have received nothing. So, we're still in the dark as to why this particular bug attacked him the way it did or what to do to keep him out of danger in the future. It will be at least four months before any kind of normality can resume. Weariness becomes a familiar companion, as I once again become responsible for all household tasks, as well as caring for a very frail and complex patient.

To add to the difficulties, the winter weather has decided to deliver relentless snow with freezing temperatures, resulting in treacherous ice underfoot. My frustration increases as I witness social media posts from selfish people praying for the snow to persist, in order to spend duvet days at home, with no consideration for those of us struggling to shop on foot or drive to hospital appointments. Having someone seriously ill in the family really does put things into perspective, and helps distinguish the genuine people from the rest. I have not appreciated the phone calls from friends and family who normally rarely keep in touch or show any interest, and I have not felt pleased to receive emails from those who usually can't be bothered, just because their morbid fascination means they want to know all the gory details.

I have appreciated the people who have offered to take me to the hospital or helped me with shopping. I am indebted to people who quietly leave milk and packages of bird seed on my doorstep without even ringing the bell, and those who send handwritten letters and cards expressing their concern and offers of kindness, as they realise I need to keep telephone lines open and would be exhausted explaining the situation over and over again.

Yes, I'm grateful there are still so many good people in the world and I thank those surrounding me with care, both near and far. But sadly, this week of hazardous weather highlights the qualities of many who just cannot think beyond themselves. I hope if they do become housebound over the weekend they don't need a doctor, an ambulance or a visit to a hospital, but if they do, maybe they'll think twice in future about what really is important when inclement weather arrives.

When conditions improve we're able visit our son's house where we're greeted by the grandchildren excitedly informing us that Mummy is having a baby. I'm not totally surprised but sadly cannot feel it is particularly good news considering the continuing disharmony, the financial difficulties and the added stress a new arrival will place upon both our son and his wife. The baby is unplanned of course, and I can't help feeling annoyed with both of them for their carelessness, but a new life should never be something to condemn, so there is nothing to do but accept the impending addition of another grandson due in July. Our son is disappointed to be expecting another boy, but consoles himself with the thought it doubles the chances of having a son who likes football.

In June my husband is well enough to travel and we fly to Menorca for a week's break. Most of our holidays in the past have been spoiled by some trauma at home and this one turns out to be no different. After a routine hospital appointment our daughter-in-law had been recalled urgently, but it seems an oriental buffet was more important to her, so she had ignored the call. Eventually, it's revealed she is suffering from pre eclampsia and in view of her other pregnancies it is necessary to perform an emergency C section. So as we sit helpless in our hotel room overseas, awaiting news in the middle of the night, our second grandson arrives in the world five weeks early and weighing just under five pounds. Thankfully, there are no complications or resulting problems, but she is advised to have no more children due to internal scar tissue and the high risk of premature births.

It will be a long time before we're in a position to take any more holidays or have any breaks from caring. Alongside helping out with our son and family, my husband's mother's deterioration continues, which entails many hospital admissions and the eventual move to a care home where she spends her last days. At ninety-nine no one can complain or feel brokenhearted, but again it's just so awfully sad to see those we care about deteriorate over such a long period of time while awaiting that dreaded phone call. It's a subdued Christmas without her but at least an improvement on the last, when my husband had been in intensive care. Painful memories and flashbacks still haunt me and fear of any further traumas is difficult to suppress. I just long to live without the fog of anxiety that seems to surround me.

Life Got Cold

April 2014

I sometimes feel really guilty that my son is an only child. Admittedly he has a half sister from my husband's first marriage and they've generally had a good relationship, despite there being an eleven year age difference. Sadly, I've witnessed friction and problems between them since he married, and as she has six other siblings on her mother's side she doesn't need his support, as he does hers. Another thing I can do nothing about, but it hurts to see the disharmony his choice of partner has caused in the family. I try my best but am only human and cannot say with hand on heart that I believe his relationship with his wife is something I feel will ever be trouble free, if indeed it lasts. I'll always support my son whatever happens but know he'd probably benefit from having a sibling he'd hopefully be able to share things with.

I feel blessed to have a sister who I consider my best friend and who has been a tremendous support for me in times of trouble. The distance between us geographically means we see each other less than we'd like, but we keep in touch on a daily basis and the times we do spend together are very precious to us both. I'm on a short stay at her house when I come across something on the internet posted by my daughter-in-law that confuses and disturbs me.

I discover photographs she has posted online of a wedding in Cambodia, with a banner displaying the year 2014 clearly visible behind the happy couple. Other photos from the occasion are of family and friends, including what looks very much like her parents who she has claimed have both died while she has been living in England. I can prove nothing and accept there could be an explanation, but feel disturbed by my discovery. I'm not generally very keen on social media sites and this is one of those occasions when I wish I hadn't looked. Unfortunately, now I've witnessed this post, which makes no sense to me, it's difficult to put to the back of my mind. I have always felt a little suspicious of her claims but have kept my thoughts to myself to avoid confrontation. This time, I can't help feeling compelled to carry out some subtle investigation.

On my return, when my son and family arrive for an overnight stop, I try to quietly discuss the worrying matter with them. I should have known better, as after all this time I am fully aware how easy it is to offend my son's wife and how she is still deeply immersed in her culture and its strange ways. Some vague explanation is given before all hell lets loose once more and as usual results in stalemate and no solution, leaving me feeling guilty and apologetic, while she sulks and ignores me. Eventually, they go out to meet friends and we look after the three children. Things calm down somewhat the following day and I just have to accept I will never understand or trust my daughter-in-law, or my son for that matter. It seems nothing will change and keeping my mouth shut a necessity if I want to avoid conflict and being condemned online.

Despite my positive experiences with the internet, I'm fully aware of the darker side of the technological world. I try to avoid disputes, political or religious debates and don't think airing your dirty laundry online acceptable, so keep away from those sort of things. My daughter-in-law however, tends to always turn to social media for attention; posting her grievances and problems for all to see and frequently attracting a lot of comments from mainly Asian readers. It has caused a lot of upset over the years, but it's not something she's prepared to stop or even modify, no matter how sympathetically she is asked. She frequently slags off her husband, her life and family here, using language I'm ashamed to read. Any criticism often results in temper tantrums and unfriending or blocking those she feels are finding fault with her and anyone else associated with them.

If we refuse to look after the children or lend her money she frequently posts streams of abuse. Her Asian followers comfort her, encourage her to retaliate and suggest Cambodian families would be much fairer, to which she responds that one day she will bring her husband and children to live there and we'll be sad and lonely old folk. I know it's all so silly and immature and I should be used to her moods, but I find it so hurtful and upsetting that we have to endure this sort of thing to try and keep the peace; that after all we've given her and done for them she can be so fickle and have no consideration for our feelings or culture. Our son is stressed and bogged down with work, seeing to the children and all that running a home entails. He is not blameless, but I don't think he has the time to be looking at what she posts online and complaining about it would only add to his stress.

I realise we will never be able to discuss anything rationally with her and it just saddens and frustrates me. I have no desire for family disputes or for them to have marital problems, quite the opposite, but I fail to see how we can continue bottling things up, papering over cracks and knocking ourselves out to help when she is just not willing to be reasonable. Seven years of this, along with other issues has made me very weary indeed. If I keep biting my tongue at this rate I'll sever it completely.

Family disputes soon have to be put on one side when all three children go down with chicken pox and my husband develops a mystery pain in his left leg, curtailing all activity. An ultra sound scan reveals his pain is caused by inflammation around his prosthetic hip joint and he awaits an appointment with an orthopaedic surgeon. After the horrendous two years of trauma and infection over a decade ago, the thought of another hip replacement is pretty daunting for all of us, but if there's no other way, then it will have to be.

After weeks of clacking around on crutches clutching hot water bottles, he goes through a small operation to remove some fluid from around the joint in an attempt to finalise a definite diagnosis and appropriate treatment. He can do little around the house or leave it very often so the extra load is making me tireder than ever and the lack of space and time increasing my irritability and feelings of despair.

Weeks later, he endures another operation which turns out to be more complicated than anticipated but successfully repairs his cracked pelvis and replaces the disintegrating cup in the prosthetic hip. He is soon back home with the familiar crutches I've now christened Crispin and Cuthbert as they've almost become part of the family. Facing another six weeks of clacking and constant company as well as caring, anxiety hangs like a dark impenetrable cloud but there is no way I can allow a full blown bout of depression at this stage, so simply have to keep going as best I can, though I'm unsure how much longer I can hold back the tide.

Once the convalescence comes to an end, life as we know it resumes, though there is little time to be carefree with helping out our son's family, the continuing disharmony, and worries over my husband's future health. It's a short-lived reprieve however, as within weeks his right knee starts to cause him severe discomfort and after a pain relieving injection he wakes the following morning unable to get out of bed. Reviewing information about the past and considering his history, a visiting doctor arranges for an ambulance to take him to hospital for investigation. It takes seven hours for the ambulance to arrive, by which time he is in agony and once more we find ourselves anxiously awaiting news of blood test results and a diagnosis.

Within days an operation takes place on his knee to clean out the joint and check for infection. He is put on an anti biotic drip, but we still don't really know what is wrong or what has caused it. There never seems to be a doctor available to discuss things with, and the lack of communication between departments and staff is painfully evident. All we are told is they think they have cleared any infection, but if not he will face another operation.

His knee is still very swollen and painful and though he is unable to come home, I already know we'll be facing yet another lengthy recovery period with the dreaded crutches, but at least he'll survive.

After spending three weeks on an antibiotic drip it's confirmed the infection still has not cleared up and he will need at least another three weeks attached to it, so there is no way he can be discharged. I don't know what the chances are of spending two Christmases out of three in hospital, but coping with another one single-handed, while dealing with the antics of a dysfunctional family and hospital visiting make for another very difficult time all round, ensuring I will never face another Christmas without a feeling of fear and trepidation.

Shot To The Heart

January 2016

I have read many self help books over the years but distinctly remember the opening line of one of them. "Life is difficult." I still feel comforted and reassured by that simple statement in a world where the majority of cliches seem to infer nothing is impossible and happiness is a straightforward condition to achieve. It helps to know I'm not the only one who finds living problematic. What is living anyway? Is it travelling the world relishing new experiences every day or drifting through monotonous days dealing with the humdrum? Everyone's concept and experience is different I guess, but to truly live do we need a positive attitude or a certain set of skills? My life over many years has been troublesome, heartbreaking at times, and virtually impossible to escape a mental state tarnished by depression. Sometimes I think my life is more of an existence; an endurance, crossing off events, days, weeks, months and years as if I'm waiting for something better at the end of it. I ponder what that says about my damaged perceptions and fragile state of mind. A lot of the time it seems to take all my strength to survive.

Admittedly, things are easier in some ways with no parents to worry and care for, though the pain of loss never goes away. Time may soften the hurt, but I don't believe it ever heals. The only thing I long for is acceptance, which still isn't easy. In the last year we've managed to survive my husband's long convalescence after spending six weeks in hospital; a long period of time when the house resembled a geriatric ward with all the medication and physical aids to help his recovery. Hospitals don't ask many questions about how discharged patients will cope at home, or the effect it may have on carers. I just hope they have completely eradicated the infection but live in fear of the next one. There appears to be no one who can explain why he keeps contracting these awful, debilitating infections and what can be done about it. This doesn't feel right or fair but there seems nothing I can do about it.

We've also survived our daughter-in-law spending a couple of months in Cambodia with the youngest child, helping out our son to care for the older two and tolerating the strop we have grown used to on her return. She admits Cambodia has changed a lot and states she won't want to go again. She seems quite appalled by the corruption and crime she's witnessed. The standard of hygiene and health care also upset her, so she's obviously become westernised in some ways. As expected, it doesn't take long after she's finally recovered from her extended jet lag before she's talking of returning again for her sister's wedding. It's wise not to ask where the money is coming from or what she intends doing with her three children, as we know from experience many of her plans and ideas turn out to be flights of fancy.

My husband is finally scheduled to receive a much needed knee replacement, sooner than anticipated, and although I have to grit my teeth at clacking crutches, wall to wall sport on television and very little space or spare time, it's a relief when it goes ahead with no problems.

We all have times in our lives when nothing seems to go right, worries and anxieties dominate our days and we hear nothing but bad news. Thankfully, there are also times when things go swimmingly, pleasant experiences dominate and life seems almost trouble free. I have memories of both, yet feel the balance hasn't been very equal and the bad times outnumber the good. I blame myself a lot and often feel ashamed that maybe my negative attitude influences the way I see things. Changing your nature isn't an easy task and after many years of accumulating bad memories I find myself almost constantly tired, nervous and stressed. My emotions have been knotted so tight, so many times over a long period, I find it virtually impossible to feel carefree or cast aside fears for the future. Maybe I wouldn't know what to do with a peaceful existence.

We survive a comparatively uneventful Christmas for once and I even joke that my husband is following the pattern of football matches in having one at home and the next away. I try to count my blessings, but it's difficult to maintain positivity or make concrete plans when there seems to always be something turning our lives upside down, but we continue to hope things will become easier as sometimes hope is all we have to cling to.

I always breathe a sigh of relief when Christmas is over and hopefully look forward to a quieter, uncomplicated time. Despite my lack of enthusiasm for the festive season I've always believed Epiphany is the date when decorations should be packed away, but for some reason I break my own rules and take them all down the first weekend of the new year.

For years my husband and I have spent Tuesday evenings with some close friends, alternating between their home and ours. Most of them are spent with drinks and nibbles, the men discussing mainly sport and my companion and I flitting from one topic to another. Invariably my husband consumes too much wine, then becomes rather awkward and argumentative and the first Tuesday of January is no different On our late arrival home by taxi he pours himself another drink and flops down in his chair. The one no one else dares to sit in. I silently wait for the predictable late night debate.

'What do you want to do with the rest of your life?' Not a question I'd anticipated.

'You know the answer to that so there's no point debating it.' He's aware I want to move to Newark, a town I've grown to love.

'Why do you want to move there?'

'Does it matter? I know you wouldn't agree.'

'Well, it's too far away from the kid's homes for one thing.'

'Maybe that proves you think more of them than me.'

'You just want an argument. I'm going to bed. My back really hurts.'

'Well, you have a doctor's appointment tomorrow. That should help.'

'I don't think there's any more help for me. My body's had it.'

The following morning, Epiphany, brings the usual apology from him and my suggestion that next time we spend an evening with friends he goes straight to bed instead of instigating pointless discussions. He later sets off to Derby where he is to collect the two older grandchildren from their first day back at school, then help to set up a new washing machine at our son's house. I always enjoy my rare times of space, but for some reason as I turn off the light in my craft room upstairs I'm thinking maybe these dark winter afternoons are not ideal for solitary activity. I prepare the dinner, a new chicken recipe my husband isn't too keen on trying; preferring red meat and familiar dishes. Time passes by and I begin to wonder where he has got to, concluding there must be a problem either with the family or the washing machine.

Time slows as anxiety rises but still after sending several texts and making a call to his mobile I try to convince myself his phone is out of earshot or he's driving, so can't answer the call. I know I'm a worst scenario type of person; understandable to some extent after all the shocks in the recent past, but suspect I have always been this way. As a child I could even see the downside of a bowl of ice cream.

I decide to have my dinner which is surprisingly pleasant, but by this time I am getting seriously anxious and just want to have him home to share the meal.

You see the scene in dramas and films and shudder, hoping against hope and dismissing the idea it could ever happen to you. But when a policeman knocks on your door you know it has. The only worst thought is that something has happened to my son or the children, but I know what is coming and back myself up against the wall.

I don't take in the details at the time, but the fact my husband is gone is all I can comprehend. I don't absorb much else apart from the policeman phoning the friends we'd only seen the previous evening and asking them to come to the house, then phoning my sister who arranges for her husband to drive her over from Staffordshire. There are many times during depressive episodes and stressful situations when I've not known what to do with myself, but the agonising pain of the reality of this situation is beyond any strategies I've attempted in the past. The night passes in a blur of uncontrollable tears and disbelief, including having to phone my stepdaughter later with the devastating news. His death had occurred very suddenly at our son's house as he was trying to install the new washer, sadly leaving our daughter-in-law to deal with it initially and unfortunately, partly witnessed by the grandchildren. The only thing we console ourselves with is the fact it had not happened as he was driving the children home from school.

I spend the next week at my sister's in Staffordshire in a distressed state, leaving my son and stepdaughter to deal with the initial formalities. There has to be an autopsy and at the end of the week I receive a call confirming it had been a cardiac thrombosis and nothing could have prevented it. I will always partly blame the initial hip replacement that went so badly wrong for my husband's death. Over the years and after multiple infections, hospital stays and operations, his activity had been greatly reduced; lack of mobility being one of the main factors contributing toward any blood clot. We cannot be issued with a death certificate until it's decided whether there will be a burial or cremation, so wanting to do things fairly I phone my son and stepdaughter to discuss this with them. There are no specific formal last wishes left by my husband, but past conversations and related funds indicate he would not have wanted anything elaborate or costly. Our son only expresses a desire to go along with my wishes, but there follows an awkward conversation with my stepdaughter which doesn't help matters and ultimately leads to further family conflict.

We cannot hold a funeral for five weeks, during which time there are many frustrating and incompetent dealings with banks, funeral directors and utility companies. I spend much of my time on the phone, tackling formalities, making arrangements and all the unpleasant tasks that are essential after a death in the family. I'm running on adrenaline, not sleeping well and reeling from one extreme emotion to another. On the whole people are kind and helpful and yet again I thank technology for enabling me to keep in touch with friends, as well as tackling business. There are also some highly spiritual moments which I know from experience are due to heightened emotions and which I hope will bind our small family together during this awful time. Maybe grief gives us a manic energy to enable us to cope, but I'm aware it will be temporary and daren't think about what may happen in the future, so cling precariously to my one day at a time philosophy.

Between meltdowns and moments of disbelief we manage to arrange a funeral but not without some friction, particularly with my stepdaughter who seems to want everything done her way with little regard for my feelings or beliefs. Neither she or my unsociable brother-in-law even ask if I am in a financial position to afford the elaborate arrangements they seem insistent upon, or offer any contribution towards the cost. My son and I are frequently annoyed and in disagreement with her ideas but feel determined to keep quiet and just get the whole awful ordeal over with. In very tough times you see the true colours of people and they aren't always the shades you prefer. I try hard not to judge, as we all react differently and vary in our values and opinions but over these heartbreaking weeks my allegiances change significantly, though thankfully, and sometimes surprisingly, some people prove to be pure gold, both close by and across oceans and it is those who hold up the much more vulnerable, flaky and frailer creature I have become.

Crash And Burn

March 2016

After a very stressful and emotional funeral which is nothing like I'd have wanted but more to appease my stepdaughter, I hope some of the heartache of loss will ease a little. I drift through the long days in a haze, though there is still plenty of paperwork and officialdom to deal with, none of it pleasant. Friends help when they can, but the reality of living alone for the first time in my life is a chilling prospect and cannot be dismissed. Becoming an orphan and a widow in the space of seven years is a heavy burden to carry, alongside the ever present anxiety over our son's family situation. Add to that the resentment simmering in my stepdaughter and it's becoming obvious to others the load to bear is nearing too much. Nights spent alone are agony at times and weekends very lonely as others carry on with their family arrangements. I try to alter any familiar routines and fill my days as best I can, although I dare not think about life ahead, which seems to offer very little. I struggle with physical health problems, battling one nasty infection after another, but I know my mental state is deteriorating as the casserole bringing neighbours taper off and my family return to their routines as best they can. My brother-in-law flies out to New Zealand the day after the funeral, but I wouldn't have expected much support from him and my stepdaughter and family barely communicate. It is purely a matter of getting through each day and waiting for a glimmer of hope in the darkness of reality. I've had some tough times in the past, but this is proving to be something far more challenging.

Alone and grieving I'm finding it difficult to even think about what lies ahead, but the one thing I know for certain is that I will have to move house, sooner rather than later. For some, remaining in their marital home brings comfort, surrounded by familiar possessions and routines a way of coping, but for me it's a nightmare. Painful memories lay like a blanket of dust over everything. I'm haunted by the house, by all the anguish endured over the years, by my choices and my mistakes. Nothing will ever be the same, the familiar taunting me with distressing, crippling thoughts and I cannot imagine things ever improving if I remain here. I have grown to dislike the area I live in intensely, but my friends and activities are here, so I initially dismiss the idea of moving to a completely different area.

Once the formalities lessen I turn my energies to slowly and painfully clearing out; systematically ridding each part of the house of possessions and furniture no longer needed, knowing that wherever I move to it will be a much more compact residence and will only need equipping with essential items for one. Disposing of someone's belongings after their death is a profoundly harrowing experience and not something I've ever wanted to contemplate doing for my partner, particularly as my husband has always been a rather untidy hoarder. I'd frequently asked him to consider the work and responsibility I'd have if he passed away, but it had fallen on deaf ears and now the massive chore is solely on my shoulders. The worst part is contemplating how on earth I can dismantle the massive model railway he's worked on for years in the loft; an area of the house I've refused to enter for several years. His obsession with steam railways has led to a huge collection of hand built models, track, books, videos, tools, as well as drawers and cupboards full of unfinished projects. It's an overwhelming, agonising and exhausting task for me to sort it all out and gather it all together in one room. I inform my stepdaughter over the phone that sadly it will have to go, and I agree she and her family can take whatever they want before it is sold. Sadly, this obviously wasn't enough for them, leading to interference, embarrassment and further disharmony. They seem oblivious to the hurt they cause and ensure more of my anchors are cut loose.

I know they are horrified when I tell them the house is going up for sale but refrain from reminding them it is me who has been left alone as chief mourner and my future plans not really their business. Time begins to crawl and I question frequently why I am still alive, left alone, heartbroken and seemingly with no purpose. Waking too early with an overwhelming feeling of loss and no incentive to continue living, attempting to find things to occupy the days and long lonely evenings, failing to find how to survive weekends when others are busy with their own families are all crippling experiences and the meltdowns increase over the weeks.

I also began to contemplate whether moving to an area I like that holds no bad memories may be a better option than staying somewhere I dislike, with far too much painful history. I start researching properties in the town of Newark; a place I'd fallen in love with on my first visit. By a strange coincidence it was due to my first mental breakdown that I'd been introduced to Newark; a place I had never visited before then. From my short spell in a psychiatric hospital I had inadvertently crossed paths with another patient on a different ward who resided in the town. After being discharged, I started to visit her with other friends and had spent many happy times there.

A later depressive period when I had turned to the internet football chatroom as a distraction had led to me forming a friendship with an anonymous man from Barnsley, where I'd studied at college many years previously. We later discovered we both considered Newark one of our favourite places and had taken the plunge to meet there for coffee, leading to a valued friendship which is still ongoing after many memorable times spent together. I had often broached the subject of moving there to my husband, but he would not even contemplate the idea. Although I feel guilty that his death now gives me an opportunity to move, I conclude my chances of coping alone are higher if I leave my home town behind and start afresh in a place I really like.

I put my own property on the market and I start to peruse the properties for sale in Newark, deciding as I will only require a small abode I should be able to find something in Newark I can afford. It's on the day I first go to view some properties that the adrenaline stops racing, the reality of all that has happened hits me like a brick wall and I know as I sit on the train returning home, that depression is travelling with me and has won the battle. From that moment on I feel terrified.

Fighting depression is not a new experience for me, but there is a depth at which it is impossible to succeed and I know I have reached it. Only once before have I hit the proverbial rock bottom; an experience I will never forget and one I hoped never to repeat.

My previous encounter ended my career. With hindsight, teaching maybe wasn't the best profession to choose for someone with negative tendencies and a propensity to depression, but I managed twenty-eight years at the chalk face with no major crises or breakdowns. It's almost impossible to feel indifferent around children and the demands of running a classroom, so there were many highs and lows, but over the years, with the support and encouragement of two wonderful Headteachers I mostly felt secure and valued in my work. Then came the boss from hell.

I had tried. I bent over backwards to please, jumped through hoops and turned somersaults in an attempt to cope with an unrelenting stream of ludicrous demands and unyielding pressures, but the new broom with steel bristles arrived with a ruthless agenda. Anything and everything residing in the school before her arrival had to be swept away.

Eventually I cracked. My symptoms do not necessarily apply to everyone who suffers, but every aspect of severe depression is frighteningly intense. The feeling of elastic bands snapping in my head as the altered brain chemicals flow, the heightened senses in the worst possible way, the inability to eat, sleep, concentrate, socialise, converse, laugh, travel or even move at times are just some of the physical sensations. But the mental and emotional symptoms are the crippling ones.

I spent ten agonising months at home attempting to claw my way out of the black hole, trying and failing to resurrect my life and ability to return to work. I just didn't believe I could stop working and still carry on living. Family and friends despaired; even the family dog seemed scared of me. But there was no hint of recovery so I was admitted to a psychiatric ward. It was one of the worst experiences of my life. I knew it would not help me in any way.

After the longest two weeks of my life I told my husband I could stand no more. We eventually managed to see the ward doctor to ask if I could be released for a weekend break.

She made no eye contact but rustled through notes before stating flatly that she didn't advise it, but if my husband was prepared to look after me and ensure my return on Monday, then she couldn't prevent me from leaving. I walked away from the hospital without a backward glance. For sure I wasn't well; far worse than the doctor was aware, but I felt certain there was no way I would return on Monday or ever again.

Two months later, a drug free cocktail of pretence, determination, support from friends and surprisingly, technology, resulted in a full recovery. I took early retirement and looked forward to a fresh start with no more hassle, teaching, medication or depression. I had found my own strategies for dealing with it and vowed it would never happen again.

We know not what the future holds for good reason. Over the years, so many times I've found myself teetering on the edge of that black hole as one trauma after another blasted my life. But somehow I have survived them all and managed to avoid falling.

But after sixteen years of coping, my strategies have backfired, my safety rope has snapped and I find myself buried deep at the bottom of the pit, unable to function.

End Of The Line

April 2016

From the moment I step into the house after my visit to Newark, every conscious moment becomes a living hell. All the familiar symptoms from sixteen years ago return with a vengeance and despite attempting every strategy I know, there is not one glimmer of hope. I cannot focus on anything apart from my own dark thoughts. Several visits to the doctor result in more and more medication I have no faith in. Appointments for bereavement counselling are not going to happen in the near future and I'm desperate for something, anything, to stop this spiral of depression I cannot control. My appetite closes down, my sleep is erratic and disturbed, my concentration out of control. The long, empty days are torture. Friends try to help, but I know ultimately only one person can get me out of this state and that is myself; a terrifying truth.

I try to keep going, attempt to focus on reading, writing, following a film on television, knitting, anything that might prove I am still capable of functioning, even at a basic level, but nothing helps. The simplest tasks, the simplest solutions to the smallest problems are beyond me. I sink lower and lower into the depths of despair and become paralysed with fear. Palpitations, sweats, the inability to relax and panic take over despite efforts to control them. I feel more alone than I've ever felt before. After so long of dancing around the needs and wants of others, always having to give so much of myself, being set free turns into a paralysing prospect. It's three months since I lost my husband, yet it seems now the world has deserted me and expects me to have recovered. Grief isn't an illness and there is no medication to cure it. Yet I know, despite the shock and loss, despite the grief and heartache, the biggest factor is fear of the depression itself. They say there is a rope ladder out of depression, one you can use to climb out of it, but I have no idea how to even reach out for the first rung.

Knowing I have instigated my own recovery in the past is now a petrifying thought. This time I cannot do it and feel there will never be a cure; the idea of living in this state with only one way out becomes unbearable. I know this illness too well. Analysing drives me crazy and provides no answers. I realise I couldn't accept the death of my husband, adrenalin had kicked in and mania took over. There was so much to do and many people around. I thought by moving house I would feel better, but then it hit me I was just running scared. Fear of severe depression returning ensured it did, and knowing how hard it is to fight just feeds its power. I have no fight left.

I stay with friends for a few days, but although it is preferable and safer to be with other people, it is not going to take the reality or the depression away, and I know returning to life alone is something I cannot avoid.

I'm aware my family is less supportive than others and their presence makes little difference. My brother-in-law is in New Zealand, my stepdaughter and family virtually ignore me and my son is busy and weighed down with his own family. His wife is due to fly out to Cambodia again with the youngest child for three months and my son plans on joining her with the other two at a later date. Friends try to help, but their lives continue the same and their conversation does not catch my attention. I resent everyone still having their lives in tact while mine is shattered. I have suffered so much heartache and dealt with such a lot over the last fifteen years and somehow coped. This time I have cracked and am being hard on myself. A crisis team visit every day, but the members differ on a daily basis, the visits are short, and suggestions of making a cup of tea or going a walk are hardly going to improve matters.

After a few weeks of what I consider agonising torture, I decide I've had enough, I will never recover from this unbearable depression and there is only one way out. I feel the only way is to escape from a life that has never seemed enough but has now proved to be too much to bear.

Most days a friend visits or takes me somewhere and it is on the last Friday in April when I ask my companion to drop me off in town as I want to do some shopping. I purchase a packet of paracetamol from every chemist in my town, where pharmacies outnumber any other kind of shop, and a bottle of gin from the supermarket. I spend hours researching on the internet how much medication and alcohol is necessary to ensure there will be no recovery. I empty all my anti depressives, sedatives, sleeping pills and the paracetamol into a bag, even hiding it outside in case anyone drops by, then dispose of all the packaging in a bin on the nearby park. I eat nothing and sit waiting for the long night to arrive.

Many think suicide is a coward's way out, but I don't consider that the truth. It takes guts to decide to end your life, even when it's agony, and even more courage to go through with it. It's considered a selfish act and I can agree with that, but when you feel so distraught and useless you can't believe anyone would want you around, you don't really think about the effects it will have on those left behind. Your self loathing is so ingrained you can't imagine how anyone could love you anyway. Verdicts frequently claim the mind of the suicidal person is too disturbed to know what they are doing, but that is not always accurate. I have thought it through and logically decided there is no other solution.

I have no idea how many tablets I swallow, but I hold a mound in my hand before taking the final step. How many times I repeat that action I don't know, but when I come round I am on the kitchen floor, though I don't recall going in there. All that comes to mind is to get in bed and sleep for as long as possible, but nothing alters and I'm awake at six in the morning. I am violently sick a few times and manage to convince the member of the crisis team who comes to the house that I am ill, don't need anything, and just want to go back to bed. It is only when a friend phones and suspects something is wrong that the details emerge and she is soon at my house and summons an ambulance. It takes a while to arrive and I am taken to hospital where my sister is already waiting. I feel deeply ashamed, embarrassed, angry and nauseous but mostly fearful, knowing what the most likely outcome is now going to be.

Back To Black

May 2016

I spend four sleepless nights in the main hospital. Nurses with stern and unsympathetic expressions initially watch my every move, even accompanying me to the toilet. I don't know what ward I am on, but I am definitely the youngest patient in the room and probably the fittest. Apart from sporadic vomiting and weakness there is little wrong with me physically, which only adds to my already heavy guilt. Throwing up is something I try to avoid and in general I succeed, but this is something else; something uncontrollable, humiliating and evokes no sympathy. The three elderly patients sharing the room are wrapped up in their own worlds of dementia, immobility and basic bodily functions, constantly irritable and demanding of the staff. They choose to ignore me unless my needs are attended to before theirs, which then results in resentment and loud complaints.

I spend my days pretending to be engrossed in colouring, completing puzzles or reading the magazine a kind visitor of one of the other patients has brought me out of sympathy, but in truth I can concentrate on nothing and the inner turmoil of the last few months is still unremitting. I remain quiet, exchange pleasantries with staff and ask for very little. A model patient in some respects, but how much can be deduced from an external facade? Inside I am still screaming and don't want to be conscious or even alive. The nights are unbearably long and sleep a rare luxury. Deprived of alcohol, nicotine or medication, barely able to eat or escape my whirling, disturbed thoughts I lay in petrified stillness like a rabbit in headlights, watching the sun rise over the high roof of the hospital buildings, the thought of yet another endless day unbearable.

I know I have to escape. I know I don't belong here. I know I can't go home. I know I will probably be transferred to somewhere else I despise. I know in reality, there is no escape.

A smiling doctor confirms my fears, suggesting a few days over the way won't do any harm and I am wheeled to the unit I swore I'd never see again by two cheery nurses who use the excuse to light up. I'd join them if I could be bothered, but even smoking has lost its appeal if not its cravings, and besides, it would probably bring on another bout of vomiting.

I cringe as the lift and its programmed, monotone announcements bring back memories I hoped were buried deep in the past, never imagining I would find myself confined inside its cold, metal walls again. Flashbacks from years ago hurtle through my distraught mind like a horror movie, alternating between fast forward, rewind and repeat. The experience has never left me it seems; memories now invading my already tortured mind.

I'm reliving the days spent languishing on a hard bed with synthetic covers, counting the spots on the curtains but never getting beyond nine for some reason, while my inner thoughts spiralled out of control. My rare movements involved essential visits to the toilet, yet even there feeling unsafe; in fear of being watched. I'd stumble along corridors to the smoking room and had to be cajoled into lifts, then herded to the dining room by staff in an effort to make me eat. I could only ever manage orange juice and ice cream.

I recall having to be coaxed to take baths in lukewarm water behind unlocked doors, feeling so petrified that rapid drying with starched, faded towels was almost a relief, yet exhausting when movement of any kind required monumental efforts. Visiting the day room with its battered domino sets, dog eared books and incomplete jigsaws but unable to focus on anything. Other patients transfixed by the television screen offering no conversation or company and nameless, faceless nurses showing little sympathy or understanding; tick boxes, targets and tea breaks their top priority. Only incidents of hysterical behaviour, attempted escapes or suicides jolted them into action. Doctors confined behind private doors; inaccessible unless you were summoned. A rare occasion when shuffling papers, mutterings about obscure drugs and offers of non existent activities were as good as it got.

Memories are fragmented and disjointed. Rooms and corridors painted insipid shades with unreliable clocks fooling already chaotic minds. Pungent odours and grating sounds. A crippled mind heightens senses in the worst way possible.

Queueing for tablets with drug induced companions, in order to escape into oblivion for a few hours. Drugs help you sleep but do little to halt the flow of altered, destructive chemicals and feelings of desperation. Evidence of their failure filled every part of the ward. A diverse mixture of damaged souls of all ages, persuasions and backgrounds engrossed in their own private hell. Burly young men suffering alcohol withdrawal, others witnessing aliens from windows or pacing the floors consumed by anger. Fragile, elderly ladies stripped of their dignity and identity by the cruel arrows of dementia. Equally as disturbing the glassy eyed, smiling youngsters institutionalised by spending so much time in confinement, victims of experimental treatments.

Now here I am, back in the place I swore I'd never see again but this time in far different and harrowing circumstances, aware walking away will not be an option.

The ward doesn't look familiar, but my arrival is equally as cold, staff rummaging though my meagre belongings removing anything they consider inappropriate; the belt from my dressing gown, plastic bags, pills, scissors, yet neglecting to notice my cigarette lighter. Half-hearted nursing care is evident from the start as I am lectured on what is and is not allowed, then dumped in a cold, plastic chair while they find me a place in one of the rooms.

This ward is one designated for the elderly, a good idea in principal, but looking around me in the television room where I've been left, it appears some of my captives are as disturbed, weird and frightening as the youngsters I'd been incarcerated with last time. I'm rigid with fear and trembling by the time a nurse appears in the doorway. It's a mammoth effort to remove myself from the chair, after the nurse insists I follow the others to the dining room.

A garbled cry drifts down the corridor, increasing in pitch and volume until it transforms into an unearthly wail. Erratic, rhythmic clattering of metal follows; a cutlery and formica overture, out of tune and threatening. I freeze on the spot. How on earth can I survive here? An inmate comes to the rescue. A tall, smartly dressed lady with large glasses, immaculate dentures and a gravelly voice.

'It's okay, duck. I'll shut them up. You'll be okay with me.'

She leads me down the corridor to where the noise emanates. The dining room. I have no interest in food or mixing with the occupants behind the door. My bodyguard flings the door open with the confidence of someone who owns the place.

'Pack it up,' she yells. 'You're frightening this lady. Get back to your room if you're going to cause trouble.'

The noise subsides and all eyes turn to examine the newcomer, a figure ripe for ridicule; pasty faced with wild hair, sporting crumpled purple pyjamas. I want to disappear, not caring where I go as long as it's away from here.

I sit in the small dining room of my new place of detention surrounded by a mixture of patients with vacant, tortured or wild expressions. I feel like a prisoner awaiting execution, but this will not be my last supper. More the beginning of months buried in a dark pit of hopelessness and terror, dismissing the idea that from darkness comes light.

Highway To Hell

June 2016

There are no spots on the curtains this time. Just a flimsy, pale purple fabric I try to conceal myself behind at every opportunity. My hard bed is lodged against a matching shade of wall I continuously stare at, rather than face my surroundings or the others I share the room with. One is the lady who'd rescued me in the corridor, who I envy for her ability to talk, laugh and care about her appearance. The others are strange creatures I don't want to be around or feel any empathy with. Outside the room things are even more scary with an assortment of shrieks, wails, abuse and angry rants from every direction. I'm trapped in a place where I don't fit, surrounded by random personalities haphazardly thrown together by circumstance. My terror only increases. Like a tortoise, I want to retreat into a shell and never emerge again.

The ward routines soon become apparent. Woken far too early by one of the patients in my room who repeatedly asks what time it is and shows no remorse for waking others with her loud chatter at unearthly hours. Soon followed by the clanging of equipment and raucous voices of staff as they enter rooms to wake patients and coax them into carrying out morning ablutions. There is little privacy in a small, drab washroom containing only a sink and a toilet shared with other occupants, but choices are restricted in this place. Once the massive effort of washing and dressing is completed, patients trudge to the dining room for breakfast. Some eat heartily and appear quite cheery, but for me eating is a massive ordeal. Forcing down some cereal and toast just to secure escape, I'm aware of the watchful eyes of staff as they fill in the necessary tick boxes to record intake and behaviour. My lack of appetite is frowned upon and misunderstood, so it isn't long before my morning ritual includes supplementary drinks; thick, lumpy concoctions, flavoured with disguised chemicals which are not optional, just like the drugs handed out to accompany meals. As soon as I can escape I crawl back onto my bed, hiding under a blanket I've brought in with me, and rarely move from there until the next dreaded mealtime at noon.

My withdrawal is interrupted by cleaners, rounds of nurses carrying out basic observations and disruptive patients demanding attention. I can never return to the sleep I wish was permanent, but it's the only way I can avoid activity and other people. Quiet periods are rare, with the more verbose and demanding patients frequently yelling, screaming, throwing things and being dealt with by staff. Alarms are commonplace; sometimes when patients on other wards are troublesome and staff need back up, sometimes when inmates attempt to abscond or harm themselves, sometimes when fire alarms are accidentally or deliberately set off by unsupervised patients.

My feelings towards other patients varies and much as I am immersed in my own personal hell, it's difficult to ignore the agony of others. It adds to my distress to witness one lady continuously pacing the corridors clutching a rag doll, sometimes distraught, hugging the doll close, sobbing as only the truly broken-hearted can. Other times she'll be overcome with anger, yelling abuse, swearing and spitting, violently throwing the doll to the floor. It generally takes two members of staff to control her, comfort her and inevitably return her to her room where all becomes quiet for a while; I suspect with the aid of an injection of some sort.

Some patients seem constantly scared and confused, others disruptive and abusive, or in their own worlds talking and singing to themselves. Evidence of the physical effects of mental illness and neglect is hard to ignore. Hair loss, overgrown fingernails, skeletal, stooped physiques, decaying and absent teeth are commonplace and I can't help my wild imagination visualising myself as some sort of festering, walking corpse in the future. I envisage occasions like Christmas, confined in the dreaded dining room with a microwaved turkey dinner, cheap crackers and paper hats, staff attempting to inject some false jollity into the motley assortment of broken souls. I foresee an insufferable future with no way out of this place and feel convinced I'll die here.

My interaction and opinions of the staff on the ward also varies. I'm sure I'm not wrong in seeing a sadistic streak in some who show little sympathy or understanding. Working with mental health patients must be a difficult career and requires a tough character but compassion and taking time to get to know individual patients should be equally essential. Some staff seem to act as if we are just numbers, all weak, pathetic creatures, incapable of intelligent thought or entitled to any opinions. I particularly dislike the mind games and condescending attitudes of some. Contrariwise, despite my poor state of mind, I recognise the kindness and concern of others; those who'll go the extra mile and try anything if they think it will help a patient. Sometimes I believe you can only understand mental illness if you've suffered it yourself, and the fact some of the more sensitive staff take sick leave when their own mental state suffers seems to back up that theory.

The doctors and psychiatrists are rarely on the scene and never visit the ward. Summoning patients to a meeting room once a week seems to be the norm. There, the professionals sit in a circle, laptops and notes on display, while they clinically discuss the patient's treatment, medication and progress, as if they aren't present. Once a week a newly hatched, young counsellor with orange hair and an air of rehearsed positivity attempts to talk with me about my condition, but I have already concluded there is no way out for me; the long road of battling trauma and depressive episodes just becoming too much, with no answer but to pray for the end.

Once lunch is out the way the afternoons are devoted to visitors and puerile activities usually organised by volunteers. The quizzes, table skittles and childish craft activities hold no appeal to me, but I do occasionally go on organised outside walks around the hospital grounds, though I often feel barely able to stand, let alone put one foot in front of the other. The sight of the main hospital building in the grounds brings on feelings of panic, as memories of past experiences with family members rear their ugly heads.

Most days I receive visitors and become increasingly uncomfortable sitting in the company of other patients and their relatives, so frequently ask to go outside with mine rather than face the disapproving looks and eavesdropping. Inclement weather leads me to taking them into any unoccupied room we are allowed to use. I know how fortunate I am to have so many caring people making the effort to visit, listen and attempt to help me in any ways they can, but I feel beyond help and it upsets me so much that I just cannot respond in the ways they want. Family visits are rare as my sister and family live away, my son and family are in Cambodia and my stepdaughter obviously disinterested and uncaring, as she never puts in an appearance. As time progresses I come to dread visiting times and feel slightly relieved when it becomes evident no one is coming, even though I have no other way of passing the agonising time until sleep.

I never feel safe or able to express my needs. A trip to the staff desk behind glass panels to ask for my phone charger, nail clippers, hairdryer or to use the washing machine become massive ordeals which I'll put off for hours, even days, in order to avoid being seen or interacting with staff. Sometimes I'm aware they ignore my presence or rush off to a supposed emergency. Whether their methods to deal with patients have any solid foundation I don't know, but at times it seems deliberate contradictions and inconsistency are employed, though I cannot understand the reasoning behind them.

I have to wash my own laundry as there is no one to take it home and do it for me. On one occasion a nurse informs me I will no longer be able to use the ward washing machine, due to the risk of cross contamination. Much as I'm ashamed to admit I don't really care about clean clothes and personal hygiene, I do realise things will need to be laundered, so have no idea how I am going manage. When my sister approaches the staff to discuss the ban on using the ward machine they deny all knowledge of what I've been told and make it look as if I'm imagining things or lying. It seems at times that attempts to confuse and misinform vulnerable patients are deliberately employed.

It's obvious my stomach problems and discomfort are a result of my overdose, yet staff insist I receive an enema and a bowel ultrasound across at the main hospital. Very distressing and painful procedures which highlight no major issues and are quite unnecessary in my opinion, only succeeding in adding to the high anxiety and deep depression.

Days and weeks pass with little variation within the ward, no progress in my mental state and only the addition of more and more medication as treatment. Sometimes at night I spit out some of the many tablets I'm issued by the nurse on the night round, as they never linger long enough to check they've been swallowed. I have no faith in their treatment and resent the fact they are issued without any explanation as to their purpose. Over time, their effects became clear as I slip into an almost psychotic state and become even more terrified, mostly of myself and the feelings of fear I am going to harm someone, which is completely alien to my nature. Physically, I seem unable to hold cutlery or coordinate my movements. My weight plummets, my self care becomes virtually non existent and my activity limited to only basics. I'm aware other patients are scared of me, their stares penetrating and disapproving whenever I am seen. Only patients unaware of their surroundings will sit with me during mealtimes and no conversation takes place between myself and others. I switch off my phone to avoid contact with the outside world and cannot respond to visitors or any staff who try to convince me it is all in my imagination.

I'm very distressed realising my son is on his way back from Cambodia and dread him visiting, fearing he will sense the evil I am convinced has overtaken me and disown me. In reality, when he does visit, though obviously shocked at the state I am in, he continues to return, relaying family news and general chit chat to avoid the painful silences. I am heartbroken and feel so guilty that I am putting him through this so soon after the agony of losing his father so suddenly, and knowing he really needs the help and support of a strong parent when his own relationship is on life support. I feel totally useless, a burden and unworthy of any sympathy.

I know the last desperate attempt at treatment for severe mental depression is E.C.T. I have undergone this twice in the past with no positive outcome and much as it is not a painful experience, it is very distressing and unpleasant. I'm aware of other patients on the ward undergoing this treatment several times a week, knowing their trip to the unit excludes breakfast before they are led from the ward by staff, later quietly returning to their rooms in a daze. I have already informed doctors I will not accept this treatment, but I guess things have deteriorated to such a pitch I am not allowed to have any say in matters. I don't recall any discussion or debates or when it is that I am first led to the E.C.T. unit feeling like I am about to face the firing squad.

Against All Odds

September 2016

I can't recall much about the first two sessions of E.C.T I've received this week, but I am aware of a very slight feeling of change. I'm not confident enough to believe I'm getting better but whatever is happening is certainly helping me to make an effort to improve my unbearable state of mind. After months of barely speaking to anyone, today I plucked up the courage to ask one of the other patients who is allowed to leave the ward to shop at the local supermarket, if she would bring me a couple of puzzle books and I've managed to concentrate enough to focus and complete some. It feels like a momentous achievement.

Electroconvulsive therapy, often known as electric shock treatment, has sometimes been portrayed as a form of medical abuse and the way it's depicted in films and television is usually very frightening. Yet many psychiatrists, and more importantly, patients, consider it to be a safe and effective treatment for severe depression and bipolar disorder. Few medical treatments have such disparate images.

ECT was invented in Italy in the late 1930s. Psychiatrists had already discovered that inducing seizures could relieve symptoms of mental illness. In truth, although strange and not fully understood, ECT is a safe and effective procedure for a variety of conditions in younger and older adults. However, there's no guarantee of success, and as with all medical treatments it carries some risks. For me, the two times I have received sessions of E.C.T in the past have made no difference to my depressed state of mind. The only things I associate with it from the past are the horrible smell of the anaesthetic and the distressing experience of coming round disorientated and realising depression is still overwhelming me.

Thankfully, this time It appears to be working. After each session I noticeably improve. I complete a jigsaw, write some notes and begin to be more communicative. I dread the treatment, the awful mask and foul smelling anaesthetic, the mystery of procedures while treatment goes ahead, and the coming round in a different room seated in a chair, wondering where I am. No one really knows how E.C.T. works or whether it will be effective, but this time I am certainly reaping the benefits and after receiving five treatments I feel I need no more. The flicker of light is burning and the brain chemicals needed to repair my dark state are obviously flowing. I am still grieving, scared, and missing my husband but there is now hope and evidence that I am no longer controlled by deep depression. As my son concludes, it's rather like rebooting a computer and putting parts back in full working order. I still wake in the night with feelings of fear and dread, in case my improved state has just been a dream, but each day things just get better and better and I can't describe the relief I feel.

It seems a strange thing to admit, but the last month I spend in hospital is one of my happiest in many years, looking at the world with fresh eyes and a clear mind. My appetite has returned, my energy levels soar and my relationships with some other patients and staff blossom. I've been given freedom to leave the ward, take long walks in the surrounding woodland, shop at the local supermarket and catch buses into local towns, as well as spending time back at home with some overnight stops. The best thing is being able to greet my visitors with a smile and see the joy on their faces now the long awaited recovery has arrived. Seeing my son and family, as well as my sister, and being able to go out for meals with them are experiences I thought I'd never enjoy again. It feels like a miracle, yet it's thanks to a bizarre treatment that may not make much sense. Without it I don't think I would have ever recovered.

Some of the more friendly staff are very interested in what I remember of the last four months and what has been going on in my head. I don't mind being a case study at all if it helps staff learn for future reference and understanding of others. It also enables me to witness the difficulties and restrictions they face with patients of all ages and types, suffering such a vast variety of conditions. I frequently chat to a variety of patients and it strikes me how most seem really decent people, damaged and broken by life and circumstances.

At the end of the month I am discharged and I leave the ward feeling I am no longer so afraid of the hospital and would be more willing to ask for help if my depression returns or deteriorates. In some ways I'm sorry to leave, as I know I'll miss the company, the easy pace, the routine and having very few responsibilities.

The only known side effect of E.C.T is some memory loss, but I haven't noticed any. There are many memories from the past and present I'd not object to wiping out, but although I can't recall every event and discussion in the hospital, I am perfectly able to recall what I can only describe as a psychotic episode and always will. It has been the weirdest and most frightening time of my life and I cannot explain why it happened. Logically, I suspect it must have been down to the cocktail of drugs I was given, but if anyone ever proves devils exist, I'll be willing to accept it could have been some sort of visitation or test from a source of evil.

I know there are many things I'll have to tackle ahead, difficulties, challenges, important decisions, and I will need to take one step at a time. Returning to the empty house, dealing with the complicated business of clearing out and preparing to leave will be painful I know, but I feel confident my clearer thinking and more positive attitude will hopefully get me through it all. One of my close friends describes it as my third life; the first being the time before I met my husband, and the second spent with him. Now I am alone and much as that prospect scares me, I know there has to be some advantages. What I don't expect or anticipate is the hurtful and destructive events bubbling behind the scenes, involving my stepdaughter and my husband's brother.

Things had become strained since my husband's death due to differences in opinions, beliefs and values, yet with compromise and respect I believed things could be settled amicably with no damage to relationships. No one from my husband's side of the family had visited me in hospital and now I've returned home I'm discovering disturbing things that have occurred during my absence. Things have gone missing and though I would never accuse anyone directly, I cannot dismiss my suspicions. Complicated and prolonged debates ensue via email which adds to my concerns, but it seems there is no way anyone is willing to discuss matters calmly face to face and my belief our relationship is solid enough to settle any matters without damage is proved wrong.

Eventually, my stepdaughter decides to cut myself and my relatives off completely and despite attempting to offer olive branches in the form of birthday cards and gift cards for her twin boys, Christmas cards and letters asking politely for the return of my house keys, she chooses to ignore me. It hurts and upsets me very much and though I firmly believe nothing is so bad it should lead to estrangement, I have to accept my views are not those of everyone. At present, I cannot allow negativity to destroy my state of mind, so I have to move on and reluctantly accept her decision.

My house is back on the market and despite the opinion of others, I still believe I will be better off and have more chance of survival if I move to Newark. While awaiting the opportunity, I am trying to make the most of my last few months, seeing friends regularly, taking a holiday with my sister and pursuing interests I've neglected during my illness. To help myself, my son and family through the approach of Christmas and the first anniversary of my husband's passing I take the family to Lapland for a week in December. It is hardly relaxing and there are difficulties with my volatile daughter-in-law as always, but as with other situations I conclude I need to resist interfering and allow them to deal with any future problems concerning their relationship.

After a few blips my house is sold and I am lucky enough to secure a small property in an ideal spot in Newark. The chaos of packing up, getting rid and moving everything to my new home is well worth the effort and it's a delightful time settling in and exploring this new area and the life I am building here. Experience has taught me nothing lasts and change is inevitable, so I'm not deluded enough to think the future will be problem free or that depression will never return, but I'm unaware how soon more dramatic events will threaten the stability I'm longing for.

Nothing Lasts Forever

March 2017

The grandkids find it a bit strange the first time they visit my new home, but they're adaptable creatures and soon get used to it. The town offers lots of parks and places of interest to take the children and I look forward to their visits. As It's quite a distance for them to travel they often stay overnight. They enjoy their bedtime routine of choosing a movie to watch, wrapped in blankets with mugs hot chocolate. Despite only having two bedrooms we manage to find enough space to sleep when the family stay over. Their mother doesn't always accompany them, claiming she's too tired or not well, but when she is here she frequently spends most of her time dozing in a horizontal position. I fear I may soon have a permanent indentation of her on my new sofa. I had hoped we'd be able to bond more and maybe even shop and chat over coffee, as the town is within walking distance for her and there are plenty of cafes and restaurants. I soon start to doubt that will ever happen, as her visits are sporadic and she seems distanced, moody and preoccupied.

The relationship between my son and his wife is still noticeably shaky and I feel it will always be this way. Much as I'm used to the periods of disharmony, the constant complaining of my daughter-in-law reinforces my belief she will never be content, no matter what lifestyle she leads. It saddens me they are both leading such chaotic and not particularly happy lives and I often feel tense when I suspect friction is brewing between them. I'm still not convinced their marriage will work out and maybe it would be better if they parted but understand the complications regarding the children and what choices their mother might make if they decided to split.

Several times in the past my daughter-in-law has been offered help and counselling by doctors who obviously believe, as I do, she has some significant mental health issues. This is hardly surprising considering her disabilities and the complexes she's developed as a result, but her narcissistic tendencies always result in her denying she has any problems; always blaming others for any of her difficulties and unwarranted outbursts. As someone with a history of mental health illness myself, I try to persuade her to accept help, despite not being convinced it will benefit her, yet knowing every patient responds and reacts to treatment and medication differently. I still believe stigma surrounds mental health and it's not my place to demand she seeks help, knowing only too well how long this can take and how frequently it proves to be ineffectual.

Despite my criticisms, I do care about her well being, and wish she'd accept the help offered, but my son's health and state of mind concern me most. He is constantly exhausted, obviously stressed and under pressure, trying to juggle a responsible job which involves a lot of driving, caring for and organising the children, as well as trying to deal with a demanding and often miserable, disabled wife. He's recently been diagnosed with diabetes type two, which is very worrying considering the health issues which can develop as a result. He has always struggled with his weight, but before he'd set off travelling ten years ago he'd worked hard to lose it. Over the years his weight has crept up and though I do not blame his wife, I know the restrictions imposed by sharing life with someone unable to walk far or take part in much physical activity is part of the problem. I also suspect comfort eating helps him deal with pressures and demands, but whatever the reasons it is now vital he tries to shed some of his excess weight. I try not to entertain the idea of what may happen should he become seriously ill or worse.

After a few pleasant months in my new abode, my daughter in law confides in me she thinks she may be pregnant, which could explain her increasing lethargy and withdrawal. My annoyance at them both for their carelessness has to be stifled, remembering all the occasions in the past when any disapproval has failed to calm tense situations. She tells me she will seek a termination, which doesn't come as a shock, as I'm pretty certain she has chosen this option on other occasions, both before and during their marriage. It's not my business to pry or judge, and what difference would it make anyway? It's worrying that she has been told to have no more children by doctors, yet seems flippant in her attitude towards pregnancies, despite the serious risks.

I try to put it to the back of my mind on the day my son is chosen to be best man at a close friend's wedding. Unlike his own, this will be a prestigious occasion, particularly as the bride to be has recently recovered from a serious brain tumour operation. The plans have been going forward over a long period of time and I am looking forward to joining in the celebrations. My son spends the evening before the wedding at a hotel near the chosen venue and his wife, the children and myself are travelling to the event in a friend's car. The friend will then look after the children while we attend the wedding, followed by the evening reception.

I notice my daughter-in-law seems in a strange state of mind, claiming she looks terrible and everyone is staring at her. This isn't altogether unusual behaviour and I assure her she looks lovely and no-one is judging her, but there is an unfamiliar intensity surrounding her. She isn't a heavy drinker but after the ceremony she heads for the bar instead of joining us outside while photos are taken and people socialise. When I return to her in the bar she does not appear to be drunk, yet is overly verbose; fluctuating between extreme affection and loud declarations that she wants to divorce my son. During the meal and speeches that follow she leaves the room and we are later approached by a guest, who informs us she is outside and needs our assistance. Not ideal for a best man who is expected to be in the midst of celebrations.

Outdoors, we discover her lying on the ground, immobile and covered by a blanket. A concerned group of guests surround her and I suspect both my son and myself are silently exasperated that she's managed to make what should be a lovely day for a special couple more about herself. We try to convince the watchers she is prone to dramatic behaviour and will be okay, but they insist on calling an ambulance. The paramedic confirms she has probably consumed too much alcohol but will take her for a check up at hospital. She refuses to go, then continues her display with added wailing, until the bystanders insist on calling another ambulance.

By this time the friend has turned up with the children who are exposed to the sight of their distressed mother horizontal on the floor. After a second refusal to go to hospital one of the staff has to drive her and my son back to the hotel where they are staying overnight. She remains there and misses the evening reception. I don't think it totally unreasonable that my son is incensed over the whole situation when he returns.

The following day my daughter-in-law later predictably posts her version of events on social media sites claiming no one in her family has helped her when she is ill and what awful people we are, as usual garnering sympathy from her followers.

The week after the wedding I spend in the Isle of Wight with my sister; a well deserved break I've been looking forward to. Towards the end of the week I receive a text message from my daughter-in-law, which includes a self made video of herself, crying and claiming the scratches and bruising she is exposing have been caused by my son attacking her. It's obvious some of the bruises are old and the scratches on her chest I suspect are possibly self inflicted for effect, but obviously it's alarming and upsetting. While I realise my daughter-in-law is a drama queen who seems to believe she is always the victim and is quite capable of lies and exaggeration, I cannot dismiss the idea that my son may have harmed her, even if not seriously. I am aware their relationship may have involved physical as well as verbal disputes in the past, but I have not heard any complaints or witnessed any signs of injury before, and feel despite her size and disabilities, she's strong and not incapable of physical abuse herself.

Part of me feels ashamed in understanding why anyone could be tempted to lash out at her, though I would never condone such actions. It may sound wrong and unsympathetic but previous research has suggested that Khmer women are very prone to threatening suicide, self harming for attention and sometimes desperate enough to report unfounded attacks. I also know from experience how volatile and unreasonable she can be and admit at times I could easily have lashed out at her myself.

I don't know what to believe. What I do know is, a six foot, well built man would never stand a chance of being treated leniently if a tiny, disabled, foreign woman ever reported what she considers to be domestic abuse. Whatever the truth of these accusations is, I know I need to approach the topic carefully with both of them and fear the outcome will be problematic for everyone concerned.

Any serenity and comfort I have gained from my new life and recent holiday is starting to evaporate, though I know I cannot allow the black clouds of depression to hover over me this time. I cannot face another battle of that kind and have to constantly remind myself, nothing lasts forever.

Prisoner Of Love

October 2017

It's my granddaughter's birthday and the family are holding a party at the bowling alley in Derby. I'm on the train returning from my break and finding it hard to concentrate, knowing a very difficult conversation will be necessary when I join them. I'm unsure how to tackle this and my anxiety increases as the train draws closer. I could well do without the hassle, but my conscience knows this is a situation that can't be ignored. On arrival, I bring my son and his wife together away from the children and ask for the truth.

My son confesses that after the wedding incidents they had become involved in a nasty row, and he had been rougher than he should have been with her. I am shocked but can tell he's immensely ashamed and he's adamant it will never happen again. I warn him that's a promise most abusers make and break, and it would be difficult for me to support him should there be any further incidents. My own marriage had been rocky at times and I know I'd suffered from some mental and emotional abuse, which I should not have endured. But physical abuse is something no one should tolerate, no matter what gender or circumstances. I feel pretty sure I would have left had it ever happened to me. I have no doubt my daughter-in-law is provocative and equally capable of abuse, but no way am I prepared to see my son sink to that level again. She stands by quietly, yet attentive, as I discuss the matter with my son, though I suspect she's thinking I am defending her and fully believing her claims that it's all down to him, which I'm sure is not the full story.

Within days she's bombarding me with texts, claiming he's abused her many times in the past, has forced her head down the toilet and pushed her out of cars. He adamantly denies these accusations and much as I cannot ignore them, I'm inclined to suspect my daughter-in-law is milking the situation and is intent on stirring up disharmony. I have always suspected she doesn't approve of the close relationship I have with my son. She frequently infers I do not know him as well as she does, and accuses me of always taking his side, which isn't true. On many occasions, sometimes at very late or inconvenient times, I have listened to her complaints and accusations on the phone and calmly tried to resolve situations, while being open to the fact there are generally two sides to every story.

Things calm down, but a seed has been planted and I find it hard to not feel tense around them and am constantly on edge, waiting for the next explosion. I worry too about the children witnessing their battles, and fear it is not the environment innocent little ones should be exposed to. I am determined I will do my best to not go down the severe depression road again but none of this helps with my own state of mind, which I'd hoped would be less threatened in my new life. It sometimes feels like some unknown force has determined I'll never live in peace.

My daughter-in-law is ecstatic when she receives notification she has been awarded indefinite stay in the U.K now she has been a resident for ten years. This means she no longer has to keep taking the Life in the U.K test, which she has understandably failed several times, and will eventually be able to apply for British Citizenship. I'm pleased for her and hope she won't need to go to Cambodia again to renew her passport, but later I will wonder if there was an ulterior motive behind her delight.

They go away on holidays to Turkey and Venice and my daughter-in-law assures me everything is fine between them now and they are happy together. It would be idealistic and childish to believe a couple of sunny vacations in idyllic locations will repair the cracks in their relationship. I do not, and it isn't long before another huge drama shatters the chances of any peace or harmony.

I'm sharing coffee with a friend at home when I notice my son approaching the front door, and I guess by now I'm programmed to anticipate trouble. He still lives in Derby and works full time in a job that takes him all over the country, besides seeing to the children and taking them to school, so what is he doing at my house so early in the day?

I let him in, noticing he looks tired and anxious, but that isn't unusual. His first words however, assure me my instincts have been correct. Words guaranteed to strike dread in every parent's heart.

'Please don't go mad Mum…' I've heard these words before, so grit my teeth.

It transpires when she had told him of her pregnancy a few days previously, it had come as a nasty shock. I wonder why she's avoided telling him until it's probably too late to do anything about it, and why she appears to have changed her mind about a termination but put those questions aside. A nasty argument had ensued and I can easily imagine the thoughts and anxieties whirling around his head. The idea of a fourth child would be just too much, though they are both to blame for creating one and should never have allowed it to happen.

I can't believe he would seriously attack or injure his wife in any way, but he confesses he had pinned her against a wall as she ranted and raged at him. Not something to be proud of for sure, particularly considering his promise not to do anything like that again, but too late now. She had called for a taxi, yelling at the driver from the doorway as she left, instructing him to take her to the police station. My son had grabbed her arm in an attempt to stop her and of course, the taxi driver had witnessed this action.

The police arrived at the house and his wife waited in their car before returning to the children, while my son was handcuffed and taken to the police station where he was locked in a cell awaiting his fate. She had been assessed at hospital but there were no broken bones or evidence of assault beyond a few cuts and bruises which could have been acquired from any source. I know her disabilities and careless nature cause her to be exceptionally clumsy, so cling to the idea that whatever he's done, though not right, is not overly serious. We discover she's also accused him of rape, something that horrifies us both and that he adamantly denies.

It had taken two nights inside that cell before he had been released on bail, with conditions that mean he is not allowed to return to his home or communicate with his wife in any way. My head now whirls with the implications. He's quite welcome to stay with me but what of the children? How will his wife, unable to drive, walk far, or get herself out of bed in the morning be able to take them to school, look after them properly, and ensure their safety and security? We both know she would never manage to see to their needs or maintain any semblance of order in their lives on her own, and this is deeply concerning. I can see my son visibly shaking from the experience of being locked up and the worry as to what is to happen to them all.

Not being allowed to contact his wife, even if he'd wanted to, is going to make any arrangements very difficult and there is no doubt in my mind she will make things as awkward as possible. There are no restrictions on him seeing the children, but being solely responsible for getting them ready and taking them to school and any outdoor pursuits has always been his role, alongside making sure they are ready for bed and prepared for school the next day. Organising shared care has to be through a family co-ordinator and the children themselves, though it's obvious they will have to stay with their mother during the week to be close to the schools, and his only time with them will be the weekends. Already, contemplating this is obviously crippling him, but there is nothing I can do apart from try to hold him up and ensure the children are well cared for when they spend time with us.

Within hours she's sending foul text messages to him and not heeding the terms, phoning him incessantly. Receiving no answer, she leaves message after message of abusive, threatening, hysterical rants. It's all very tragic and serious and

I can't see any way they can continue to have a relationship, but the children have to be top priority.

And so my relatively quiet, new life is shattered and the weeks leading up to Christmas just one long round of cooking, pot washing, shopping and clearing up. I suspect the washing machine may also be on the verge of a nervous breakdown with laundry overload. Nights sleeping on the sofa to ensure the children have a good night's sleep don't help but no way are the social workers, child protection, solicitors and family liaison officers involved going to have one chance of accusing my son and myself of not looking after the children well. Tired just doesn't cut it, but I will tolerate exhaustion as I iron their uniforms on Sunday evenings, ready for school in Derby the next day. I will ensure when they leave the house at six the next morning they are perfectly turned out and organised, even if it depletes every ounce of energy I have left.

Abusive and nonsensical text messages continue to be sent to my son and the oldest child at all hours of the day and night. It's so unacceptable that she is allowed to continue in this way, while my son is banished from his home and not breaking any of the restrictions he is under. Sometimes he'll block her from calling or texting, but we need to keep some evidence of her behaviour for future reference. I can see his own mental state is under threat. I discuss with him how the authorities have little idea or information regarding their characters and relationship, only seeing a giant of a man accused of abusing a tiny, disabled woman and coming to the obvious conclusions. In time, I assure him, the truth will out and he will be the one seen as the better parent and human being, but for now he's an emotional wreck, terrified of the future and broken hearted at not being with his children enough. Of course I'm disappointed and upset he has allowed himself to land in this situation, but at the same time I hate to see him in this state. His life is more important to me than anything else, and I believe somehow that galvanises a strength in myself to keep going and give as much support as I can.

Although this may not be the new life I envisioned I am determined I will not be broken again.

Walking On Broken Glass

December 2017

My son is working in Doncaster when he receives texts from his wife claiming she is bleeding heavily and needs help. She has attached photographs as evidence, and I confess I initially tell him to dismiss them as she's probably just attention seeking, and we know there's always an excess of tomato ketchup in the home she could utilise to back up her claims. I am proved wrong when a paramedic contacts him to say he is taking her to hospital and my son will have to pick up the children from school. He returns to Derby and brings the children to my house while we wait for news of their mother.

We discover she's lost the baby she was carrying so is to be detained in hospital. Of course, she blames my son for the miscarriage, even though he's not been anywhere near her and I admit I feel even more guilty for suspecting she's taken or done something to bring on the loss. In some ways I'm saddened I'll not see my unexpected grandchild, but it's for the best considering the situation and what strains another child would have created.

She demands to see the children while she is in hospital, my son having to drive them there after long days working and seeing to their needs. She seems to have no notion of the seriousness of the situation, even requesting he brings in a takeaway meal for her. Not wanting to cause friction or hassle for the children, he obliges but draws the line when she expects him to collect her dirty washing to launder. After a few days she is discharged, returns home and continues her tirade of abusive texts and calls. It worries me that she's deemed fit enough to have the children back for a few days before Christmas when the schools have broken up. While the children are with her, she sends texts from her daughter's phone pretending to be her, making statements inferring the children want to be with their mother, not us. Even in the midst of chaos and disaster she is capable of exercising her devious, spiteful side.

Christmas is hardly relaxing as we all go down like dominoes with an awful virus. Even my cat decides to join the competition for sympathy, requiring several expensive visits to the vets, but we all survive and do the best we can under the circumstances. What another year will bring is not something we want to contemplate, but it's obvious to all, it is not going to be an easy one again.

Early in the new year we struggle through the second anniversary of my husband's death and the eleventh wedding anniversary of my son. We could never have foreseen the events dominating our lives during this painful weekend.

The court case regarding the accused assault is due to take place later in January and I'm aware just how much this is playing on my son's mind. He is seeing a solicitor for advice and sharing with her the abuse and actions of his estranged wife. He still feels, probably justifiably, that he is viewed as a bullying reprobate and his wife the frail victim.

We know she isn't coping well with the children and it's now causing concern with the authorities involved, and the school. We know there are days they don't attend and other times when they are late, or arrive unaccompanied in a taxi. The abusive texts and calls continue; some now directly to me, asking why I'm not helping her. The children report disturbing things they have seen and heard in her care and we know at times she is deliberately not answering the door or phone when Social Services call. Despite living in England for ten years she has little understanding of our legal system or the complicated procedures involved in criminal offences and judicial procedures. In Cambodia, men can pay to become a member of the police force and are often bought off by those accused of offences. It's hard for her to understand her accusations are not being taken at face value and it isn't such a simple matter as she obviously thinks. I suspect she believes her allegations should send my son straight to jail for life, enabling her to have the children to herself with no more contact. I can't help but think her timing rather suspicious as now she has indefinite leave, she will no longer need a visa or the help to acquire one to remain in this country. Is it reasonable to question whether securing a life for herself here is what their relationship has all been about, or is my vivid imagination and negativity out of control?

Before all this kicked off my son had organised, booked and paid for her to take a three week break to Cambodia. If she now carries out her plans she will miss the court case and be unable to give any evidence, but I doubt she fully understands the implications of that either. One day she will tell everyone she is still planning on going, the next she isn't, but I'm pretty sure she'll go, as there has rarely been a time I believe she has ever put the children or anyone else before herself. The police warn her that if she does go, the children may be taken into care, though hopefully that is in an effort to persuade her she needs to be in court, or the whole ordeal will just have been a farce and a waste of time and investigation.

She continues to be very difficult and vicious regarding access to the children and the problems she has created. We have quite a collection of foul, vicious texts and messages she has sent, as well as evidence of continuous lies. She is proving more difficult for the authorities concerned, frequently lying and swearing at them when they try to interfere or ask questions she doesn't want to answer.

At the same time she begins sending food she's cooked for my son via the children, which I would have refused to eat for fear of what may have been added to the ingredients. Alarm bells are warning me she's now trying to manipulate him in order to secure any favours and money she may need after her trip. I try to remain tolerant, though I fail to see a way forward or how I'd handle having her back in our lives. I'm aware my son has inherited my sensitive nature and sense he's softening, and though I know it's not my decision, I fear he may be sucked back in. Surely there are limits to what he'll endure? I realise the children's security and welfare are the most important issues and know a break-up of their parents isn't ideal, but is there a solution which can be worked out with as little disruption as possible? If there is, it eludes me and my fear for the future increases on a daily basis.

As predicted, she travels to Cambodia, leaving the children, the whole sorry situation and the legal case behind her. I imagine she'll spend three weeks sitting on a beach, sipping cocktails, with little thought of her children or the mess she's left behind. Part of me hopes she won't return, but I have to consider the children's feelings. At least it gives my son a chance to return to the home with the children for the three weeks she's away. This has to be done through a court application and thankfully they are prepared to deal with the assault accusations at the same time, concluding it isn't worth another appointment with the supposed victim absent from the country. Due to the taxi driver witnessing him grabbing his wife when she'd made her initial trip to the police station, he is advised to plead guilty to common assault, which results in a hefty fine plus fees, but at least he is now free of any charges and will be able to ensure the children spend some peaceful time in their own home, allowing him to focus on his work and activities without any hassle from their mother.

I've grown used to their strange and volatile relationship, the idle threats, the angry outbursts and the periods of disharmony, followed by temporary truces but after being subjected to weeks of hell caused by her and enduring abuse with no substance, I am shocked to discover he is contemplating picking her up from the airport when she returns.

Maybe I'm an intolerant and unforgiving person, but I can't excuse her for all the lies, problems and anxiety she has caused. My son is not blameless, but he is basically a decent person, whereas she has confirmed she is a deeply unstable, selfish, vindictive character, unwilling to admit her faults or accept any help for her mental state. I have made allowances for her, understanding the anger she feels and the complexes she has developed as a result of her tragic background, but I'm not sure I have the necessary emotional tools to forgive and forget. I wish I had.

Can I return to lending her money, tolerating her mood swings and unpredictable behaviour? I have the feeling my son will relent and go back to her and a very tough life. It will be his choice and not my place to interfere. I understand he does not want the children to be upset or become involved in custody battles. I appreciate how difficult and heartbreaking it would be to walk away, start over and not be with the children he adores at all times. I share the fear that she could somehow manage to return to Cambodia with the children, but my heart bleeds to think he will tolerate the way she treats him and the risk of another episode like this one, which I am pretty sure will happen in time.

Voicing my thoughts and fears has become difficult, as I know I must allow my son to make his own decisions and try to stand by him whatever choices he makes. But like a computer, my brain starts to show signs of overload and should my ability to process these thoughts and fears exceed my ability to cope, then I'm aware panic attacks will begin. When the brain keeps processing messages of fear, thoughts become so scattered that normal functioning is impossible. It's a fine line I'm walking on, but I will do my best to keep my balance in order to be there for my son, whatever may happen in the future.

Playing With Fire

March 2018

As I feared, my son is taking the children to Manchester airport to meet their mother. I have no idea what sort of frame of mind she is in or how things will pan out back at their home. Everyone, including the solicitor, has advised him not to take her back, but realistically, he could hardly change the locks, they both need somewhere to live and he cannot afford to rent two properties. Optimistically, he thinks maybe she'll have learned she can't get what she wants by making false accusations and will make more effort to mend their relationship, but my old, cynical head very much doubts that anything will change for the better.

I know all about the complexities of a difficult marriage from experience and I also know how hard it would be to walk away. Part of me feels despondent, remembering the better family times in the past and the belief that I had built some sort of meaningful relationship with my daughter-in-law. But the abuse she has poured on me for no reason whatsoever is unacceptable and I can't erase the hurt the vile messages I've received from her has caused. Having said that, she is the mother of my grandchildren and now my son is back with her I find myself in a very difficult position. The whole saga is surely doomed to lead to a lot more angst and heartache.

If it is the only way I can maintain a relationship with my son and grandchildren I know I will have to make allowances and at the very least tolerate her. There are days when fragility dominates, fearing my own tentative grip on life is slipping again, but from somewhere comes the quiet courage to carry on, be prepared to help him out where I can and just hope the future will be less problematic than I believe. My son needs me and I need him and the children in my life. It would be impossible to carry on without them.

As expected, once they are back at their home in Derby things become very quiet on the communication front and he only sends me snippets of news regarding the children and his work. I don't know if he feels embarrassed because he has taken her back against everyone's advice, or if he is avoiding conflict, as he is perfectly aware I would find it hard to welcome her back in my life.

Social workers, child protection and other professionals will be involved for a while and I'm not sure she'll be able to deal with all this or agree to any plans suggested to her. Ultimately, it's their problem and they need to sort out the future for themselves. I don't want him treading on eggshells around her or suffering for the sake of the children. I feel pretty convinced there'll be further incidents before long which makes me nervous, but I have to try and step backwards for a while. Surely I'm entitled to a life of my own at some stage.

Over the next couple of weeks I see little of my son or the children but do speak to my daughter-in-law when she phones. I'm not sure why she decides to call me but suspect she feels it necessary to prove to my son that I am not capable of ignoring her. I speak civilly but emphasise we need no more hassle, and they must sort out whether they are going to make a go of it or decide to split up. She assures me she is willing to accept a divorce if that is what my son wants, but I know nothing will ever be as straightforward as that with her. In the past simple matters like how long he spends in the bathroom have turned into major issues.

It's a Friday evening when I receive a text from my son. He informs me his wife is behaving strangely and he doesn't know what to do. He doesn't go into detail, but I can't settle to anything afterwards and daren't phone to ask in case it causes any further escalation of problems. Eventually, he calls and tells me she is accusing him of all sorts of things that make no sense. I manage to speak to her, but it's obvious she is very agitated, accusing him of stealing money from his workplace and hiding it in secret accounts. When I suggest that is something he'd never do she puts the phone down on me. I wait and wait but there is no more communication. I send several texts, but there is no reply and now I'm feeling extremely worried, knowing sleep is not an option. Time stands still as I wait in a cowering daze for some form of communication.

Finally, I receive a phone call from the police. They inform me my son has been arrested and my daughter-in-law sent to hospital and ask if I can fetch the children. I gave up driving years ago, have no car and even if I had would have been well over the limit. It's an agonising wait as I sit contemplating what the hell has happened and trying to compose myself for when the police arrive with the children. They knock on my door at three in the morning carrying the sleepy children, hurriedly hand them over and give no details as to what is going on or what I am supposed to do to find out. Thankfully, the children aren't disturbed when I tuck them all in bed and try to catch some rest myself.

The next day is a very difficult one. The children have arrived with no change of clothes or toiletries, I have little food in the house and cannot leave to shop. Eventually, a policewoman phones to tell me my son will be released later in the day after investigation but is not prepared or able to give any further details. Thankfully, the children aren't overly distressed; sadly their lives have involved far too much disruption in the past and I guess they are used to it in a way and are quite at ease in my company. Keeping my own anxieties and fears in check isn't so easy, especially as the day wears on and there is no more news from my son or anyone else. Eventually, I manage to secure the phone number of the police station where he is being held to ask how much longer they intend keeping him there. I'm informed there's been a further incident and he's been rearrested, so is still unable to leave the police station. No details are available, though I am assured he will be allowed to leave at some stage; hardly words that offer any reassurance.

It's well after midnight when my son finally arrives, looking exhausted and distraught. His first words, ' I've done nothing wrong,' mean I have to reserve any judgement until he relays the whole story, and hopefully it will be the full truth.

For no apparent reason his wife had threatened to call the police and the eldest boy had hidden the telephone for fear of a repeat incident. Heartbreaking for a young child to hear and take such an action upon himself but not enough to stop her. She'd gone to a neighbour's house and there made a call to the police, accusing her husband of assaulting, raping, poisoning and trying to kill her, as well as stealing money, fathering a baby after an affair and hiding cameras in the house. I'm surprised she didn't throw in terrorism and high treason for added effect.

Due to the incident in the past the police had to arrest him, though I doubt they believed much of what she was saying. We have no idea why she has been sent to hospital or what the outcome of that is, but my son is bewildered as to why she is behaving this way. She may have been a difficult character in the past, with many complexes and issues, but this is something unfamiliar and absurd. The only explanation we can think of is that she has taken some sort of drugs without his knowledge.

She must have been discharged from the hospital pretty swiftly, as the reason he'd been held further by the police was a second call from her at home, informing them she'd found a parcel containing a sachet of drugs my son had received in the post. In reality this was a packet of Borax, a substance used to mix with the slime his children enjoy playing with, which he'd ordered online and had arrived in a box from Amazon. A ridiculous allegation, an annoying waste of police time, and only adding more stress to the whole situation as the police had to wait for a laboratory test on the powder before he could be released on bail.

So here we are, back in the same situation; my son living with me and the children being shunted between their mother and us. This time there is no going back and it has to be the end of their relationship. My son refuses to answer the many abusive calls and texts she continues to send and our concern over her behaviour increases on a daily basis. There are many decisions to be made, including whether he finds a new residence or she moves out of their rental property and he is allowed to return. It's heartbreaking to think he will only see his children at the weekends and this will affect where he chooses to live in the future. A future that seems destined to be extremely difficult and problematic, and constantly dominating our thoughts. The prolonged anxiety feels much like being hooked up to an electric fence; not enough voltage to kill but sufficient to keep things very uncomfortable. The unpredictability of life continues and I can't help wondering if I'm destined to never find the peace I have longed for over such a long period of time.

Not A Second Time

April 2018

Although I was apprehensive about living alone I had convinced myself there would be some advantages, one of them being only needing to shop for one. I envisaged having the time and freedom to choose what I wanted without considering anyone else's preferences or lugging heavy bags home. I've hardly had time to adjust before the latest troublesome episodes and now that is no longer an option. It's back to planning meals for a family, shopping for children's tastes, spending too long in the kitchen and pots piling up in the sink. On the other hand, being busy and considering the needs of others doesn't allow too many opportunities for introspection or contemplating imponderables.

I'm in a supermarket aisle debating over shepherd's pie or sausage and mash when I receive a phone call from Social Services asking if I can fetch the children from Derby. They explain their mother needs to attend hospital for an assessment. She has obviously caused some concerns which is a good thing, but there is no way I can travel to Derby to fetch them so my son has to return from Goole where he is working that day to collect them and bring them to my house. Within hours she is phoning to demand they are brought back, so obviously, her visit to whichever hospital has resulted in no action and we are doomed to continue living on a knife's edge, waiting for whatever her next ludicrous outburst will entail.

While it's difficult for us all living with these arrangements and particularly unsettling for the children, we are increasingly worried about their mother's strange behaviour. Whatever is wrong with her we have no idea; paranoia and psychosis don't even touch the sides. A multitude of incidents make for a disturbing time as she continues to make phone calls to the police with added accusations, tries to convince the school my son isn't allowed to collect the children and sends all sorts of weird texts accusing us of trying to kill her. When the children stay with her they report she is obsessed with taking apart the television, the computer, the lights and their technological devices, insisting there are cameras hidden inside them.

On one occasion when my son goes to pick up the children, parking nearby the house to avoid any contact with her, the eldest child struggles to the car carrying the television after their mother has refused to have it in the house any longer. This is becoming too worrying and my son feels compelled to contact Social Services expressing his concerns for the children and suggesting his wife needs help of some kind. They agree to pay her a visit.

When they arrive at the house, a taxi carrying his wife and eldest child pulls up outside. On this occasion she cannot pretend to be out or refuse to open the door and she lies when she tells them a friend has been looking after the two boys, who in truth have been left alone in the house. To some extent it's understandable we are not informed of any action, recommendations or advice she is given by service providers, yet it's also frustrating to be left guessing.

The children break up from school for the Easter holidays, which means they spend more time staying with us. Disturbing incidents continue, with an abundance of frightening and baffling incidents involving the children's mother, too numerous and complex to describe. It's perfectly obvious to us she is deeply unstable, incapable of looking after herself or the children properly and in need of professional help, but nothing we feel concerned about results in any action being taken. We know she is capable of presenting herself to suit the occasion, so can only assume the powers that be are being exposed to her better side, and in their eyes we are just being malicious for making accusations against her. She swings from wanting my son to give her another chance and declaring she never wants to see him again on a daily basis and appears to have no idea of the confusion and chaos she is creating. The children are witnessing her bizarre behaviour each time they stay with her, often returning with broken phones and tablets after she's attempted to take them apart, so it's difficult for us to relax or avoid feeling worried whenever they are in her charge.

Eventually, my son is cleared of all charges against him and his bail is lifted, so thankfully that is one less problem. He looks at rental properties in many different areas before eventually deciding it will be easier to secure a lovely property on an estate close to my home. In theory their mother will take them to school in Derby in the week and he will collect them at weekends and other opportunities, as well as school holidays.

Only a few days after he's secured the rental, when he is all set to leave for a week of work in London after dropping the children off at school, he receives a phone call to say their mother has been admitted to hospital so he has to abandon all plans, pick up the children from school and return to the empty house in Derby. We gather it's a psychiatric ward she's been admitted to so what will happen next we have no idea. My son discovers the house is in such a state he cannot bear to stay there until he's sorted it, so they return to mine for a few days.

When we are informed she's been sectioned and will be detained on a psychiatric ward for at least twenty-eight days it changes everything. We don't know the details, but my son is told not to take the children to see her, although she does keep phoning them. He is granted full care of the children and it seems likely their mother will only be able to see them under supervision, in time. It's all very sad and certainly not what we want, but it has been obvious to us for a long time that she has severe mental health problems and we can only wonder why this has not been dealt with before now. Possibly her previous visits to hospital had resulted in her being asked to be a voluntary patient and she had refused but it's distressing to think she has been allowed to have the children for so long without any action being taken. Whatever problems she has need handling by professionals and we can only hope things will improve, as it would be very distressing for her not to see her children and unfair on them too.

What the outcome will be is still very uncertain and there is little point predicting, but the focus has to be on the future of my son and the children. He clears and cleans the house they had been living in and moves to the rental close to my home. We had not known the children were going to be in his full time care, so it now looks likely they will have to transfer to different schools which will be upsetting and a big upheaval for them, but It's a fresh start for them all and I can only hope it will be for the better.

Although I have always feared his relationship would never be a success story, I could never have predicted the series of events leading up to this. I wish things could have ended differently, but now he has no choice other than to leave her behind and focus on a new life. I just hope and pray we can all cope with it and things may just settle into a more peaceful time. Despite all the hassle and conflict, we live in hope their mother will receive appropriate treatment, be able to cope and be reasonable, in order to maintain a relationship with her children. Only time will enable us to see a clearer picture for the future and we can only hope it will bring some stability and calm to what has been another very tumultuous time.

Moving On

November 2018

My dream of visiting America, homeland of my father and place of my birth, finally came to fruition back in 2009 when some close friends, who have a son living across the pond, invited my husband and I to join them on a transatlantic crossing to America. Although it proved expensive and took a lot of planning, it turned out to be an experience I will always remember with great fondness. I shed copious emotional tears when the ship docked in Manhattan and the Statue of Liberty came into view as the sun rose in all its glory. My husband and I repeated the trip with our friends three more times in the years that followed, exploring many and varied parts of the country and meeting relatives and friends. Memories I now treasure.

I didn't think I would ever see America again after the loss of my husband, which saddened me a great deal. Neither did I think I could ever handle a long haul flight, but I've just arrived back at Heathrow after a month long stay in Arizona. Our friend's son and family are now living there and I joined them for this latest trip. It was a very different experience to previous ones, staying in one location and spending more time alone, but I'm grateful I've had a break away from all the trials and tribulations at home and longing for a stress free time now I'm back.

Contemplating a peaceful return is short lived when I receive a phone call from my son before I've even left the airport. I discover he's been suspended temporarily from his job. He has worked with the company for a long time and has a solid reputation as a professional and successful employee. However, it transpires a complaint had been made to a housing officer in Derby from one of her service users. The complaint involved domestic abuse and it doesn't take much working out to realise who is behind it. Knowing nothing of the situation the housing officer had taken the claims seriously and reported them to my son's employers without looking into any background information. His employers, despite knowing the circumstances and all my son has gone through, insisted they had to follow procedures by suspending him prior to investigation. Of course, he didn't want me to know about all this while I was away, so refrained from telling me. I'm shocked, though it doesn't completely surprise me that his now ex-wife is still determined to disrupt our lives. She was discharged from hospital a couple of months ago and it's been obvious from the start of her release that she's not prepared to move on or let go of her grudges.

Things have definitely improved for my son and the children since they moved to the their new house on a lovely estate not far from my home. It turned out to be a perfect choice; aesthetically pleasing, with lots of green spaces, excellent schools, access to major routes and the chance to make many new friends. We hoped a fresh start for himself and the children would bring some much needed peace and harmony.

Life has been calmer, though even from a psychiatric ward his wife had continued to cause trouble and interfere with their lives. In an effort to prevent him having custody of the children she had told a visiting social worker he had sexually abused her daughter. As a result, the child was subjected to the "good touch, bad touch" talk at school; something she found very embarrassing and which angered us all.

On another occasion she contacted the police after phoning the oldest boy, asking him for their new address and then reporting my son had left the children alone in the house, when he was actually only outside in the garden.

Although she persisted in telling the authorities she intended taking my son to court and gaining custody of the children, insisting she is not suffering from any mental health issues, a tribunal at the hospital refused to lift the sectioning and advised against the children visiting her until they could arrange for professional supervision during visits.

My son has made a lot of mistakes and I'm perfectly aware he isn't blameless, but no way is he guilty of all the things she continued to accuse him of, including stealing her money, refusing to let her see the children, sending her abuse and hiding cameras in the house. We didn't know how her lies were perceived by professionals, as we're aware she is capable of changing her manner to suit the audience and probably convinces them she is the innocent victim. During the time she was hospitalised I watched my son deal with running a home and all it entails, care for the children while managing a full time, responsible job and remaining calm and distanced from the continued abuse. Despite his mistakes, I can't help but feel proud of him and how far he's come since the start of the problems.

All three children became more and more reluctant to visit their mother in hospital, but we ensured she saw them whenever possible and just wished she'd be reasonable over the break up. So many couples who decide to part do so in a mature and amicable way these days, and it's hard to conceive why she cannot accept their relationship is over and agree to share responsibility for the children in a civilised way. Sadly, it seems this will never be the case, which is only making matters worse for herself, though she obviously doesn't see it that way.

The incrimination and rebukes continued throughout the following months before she was finally discharged from hospital. We have never been allowed to find out about any diagnosis, treatment or follow ups that may have helped us understand her more. When my son had cleared the house they'd shared in Derby he'd discovered several prescriptions and hospital appointments that had obviously been ignored, alongside a report from one of her previous hospital visitations which identified amphetamines in her bloodstream. It annoys me to think those dealing with her must have been aware of this, yet still allowed the children to be in her care at this time, while my own home and living situation had been subjected to scrutiny.

She received a great deal of support from various services as they found a suitable social housing apartment for her and helped with her finances and official requirements. My son had kindly stored a lot of furniture for her when he moved house, but of course there were complaints and unreasonable demands on her part. All in all, she has had every opportunity to start a new life of her own and agree to taking some responsibility for the children, though it would be advisable to take things forward slowly.

But true to form there is no gratitude, rational behaviour or escape from her fickle abuse. The accusations continue and it seems obvious to us there are still issues with the state of her mental health. However, any concerns we express to those involved are dismissed, and we have the impression they conclude we are just being antagonistic.

She persists in turning to social media sites to air her grievances. We have no desire to follow her on websites or be involved in her attacks, but it becomes necessary to keep an eye on her activities to protect the children and see how far she is going to take things. She is now claiming to be in a relationship with a famous Hollywood actor; something we initially consider must be a joke, but over time we realise she is seriously convinced about. Very personal and quite disgusting videos posted online regarding her supposed involvement with the actor are disturbing to say the least and add to the concerns of leaving the children in her care. We do agree to take them to a family meeting centre in Derby where we do not have to see her, yet it allows her time with the children under supervision.

Included in her posts are photos and comments about her parents in Cambodia, who appear to be alive and well. Although we cannot prove she has lied about both of them dying in the past, it seems pretty likely and we are forced to consider how many other things she has told us about her past are untrue.

When she posts a photo of my son with all his details, accompanied by foul and serious allegations against him as if he's an escaped convict on the run, he is forced to report it. Although her actions are not direct communication, it necessitates a visit to the police, who agree the posts are a breach of the injunction and confirm they will visit her and issue a warning. If she does it again she could be arrested and possibly imprisoned. But how can anyone check on her online activity when she can join any site, using many names, then make them private and block people? We have little idea of the full extent of her online activity, or what she and any who are reading her posts are capable of, so it's difficult to feel fully relaxed.

Their break up is in the past now and though it will always be remembered as a painful time, we have moved on, accepted changes and hopefully learned from the experience. My son has finally detached himself from any emotional blackmail he has surrendered to in the past and concentrates on his future with the children. He is aware he should not have rushed into marriage but I would never say, "I told you so." He has expressed regret and sometimes feels he's wasted ten years of his life, but I remind him he has three beautiful children, we are merely human and all make mistakes.

If only his ex-wife would do the same, for her own sake and to be properly included in the lives of her children. Despite everything, we both feel sorry for her and all she is missing out on, but it is out of our hands. Until she approaches things in a sensible, mature way it is impossible to leave the children unsupervised in her care for any length of time. But will that day ever arrive?

Turning Tables

August 2019

After my first long haul flight to America with friends, I doubted there would ever be another, but never dismiss possibilities, as I'm well aware life can take unexpected twists and turns, both good and bad. I've just survived a second long haul journey, but this time I'm witnessing the manic activity at Bangkok airport. It all feels very surreal, bizarre and initially nerve-wracking. I have never anticipated or particularly craved a visit to Asian soils, but there's no turning back now as I face several weeks with my son and his children travelling around Thailand.

We've survived over a year without any major issues and have managed to establish a pretty stable and pleasant routine for the children. They are all happy in their new schools, have many friends and enjoy a much more peaceful existence. It's hard work for my son, now working for a different company, which involves a lot of travelling, but he copes and I help out where I can.

Sadly, the mental state of his ex-wife still causes a lot of concern and her aggressive abuse continues, though more sporadically. There are times when she makes little contact yet seems to spend more time posing for videos to post online along with the continuing news of her affair with the Hollywood actor, including that she is pregnant by him. She claims she will be taking the children with him to America but all this is sheer fantasy, which we suspect may be instigated by drug abuse, though whatever the reasons we still feel she isn't mentally well and needs help but are not in a position to interfere.

Ultimately, my son has to take out an injunction against her to ensure that should she continue to ignore rules and cause problems he will be able to report it directly to the police, though this is hopefully a last resort. It seems she can still create major trauma and massive problems without even being present in our lives and there are no lengths she won't go to in an attempt to cause disruption and destruction. So much effort has been put into trying to be tolerant and reasonable, but it appears she can't or won't respond to anything in a positive way.

We do not want to express any criticism or concern to the children about their mother, but there are times when he has to check their phones to see what messages she is sending to them. He continues to drive them to Derby on alternate weekends to see their mother at the family centre and eventually allows them to stay overnight with her at her apartment. It causes anxiety, but it only seems fair to allow them to have a continuing relationship with their mother, providing she looks after them appropriately and they don't return distressed. However, there are times when she doesn't want to see them or demands to change dates to suit her and visits have become very erratic.

We're pretty sure she will be aware we are visiting Thailand and the reasons why. No doubt she'll be fuming, attempting to find ways to ruin plans and ranting on social media, but these things aren't foremost in my mind.

Initially, my son informed me that although he doesn't relish the idea of being alone, he never wants to marry again, but like other things he's been adamant about in the past, I wasn't going to take his statement at face value. Besides, there's always the thought that maybe life is mapped out for us in some way and we have no way of predicting the future, despite any plans we may nurture.

Despite his insistence he'd remain single until the time was right, we're in Thailand to celebrate his engagement to a Thai lady. I don't ask about or comment on his reasons but suspect he feels more comfortable with oriental women, particularly as his children have obvious Asian genes. It is not my place to judge and as long as he's with a decent partner who makes him happy I don't care what colour, nationality, age or gender they are.

I have kept my reservations and scepticism to myself, believing him capable of making his own decisions and hopefully be more cautious about future relationships. Naturally, I'm concerned he's again entangled with a foreign girl he's only met a few times, but at least this one is able bodied and comes with no baggage.

Despite my cynical head and multitude of concerns I was quite impressed when the young woman concerned travelled alone to England to meet the family earlier this year. The fact she'd never left Thailand before, was capable and willing to do so and accepted my son with the addition of three children suggested she was hopefully honest, mature, capable and not using my son for her own advantage. The visit went well, erasing some of my apprehension and I could sense a genuine warmth and compatibility in their blossoming relationship. However, I don't think I could ever feel totally convinced any relationship will work out after all the pain and hassle from the past but maybe that's my problem and not something I need share. I keep my reservations and worries to myself.

After my initial panic attacks brought about by witnessing the frenetic, chaotic way of life in Bangkok, I start to relax and overcome some of my nervousness at being in a totally different environment. I don't enjoy all the new experiences, but it's an interesting trip to say the least and good to spend a prolonged time with my family. We travel to several different locations, some very beautiful and the sunshine, scenery and balmy evenings are very much appreciated.

My son's soon-to-be fiancee works in a government office during the week, so can only join us at weekends, but takes time off for their engagement ceremony. It takes place in a rural, unspoiled part of the country, where her family live and she grew up. It's a strange, surreal experience and not something I could ever have imagined myself doing, but despite feeling overwhelmingly conspicuous and out of my comfort zone, it proves to be an occasion filled with tradition, generosity, love and laughter. Meeting her family and seeing where she has been raised is something I appreciate as it helps with understanding her background and family circumstances.

Back in England, although there is never a guarantee relationships will work out, I try to be more optimistic, as knowing much more about my second daughter-in-law and her upbringing will hopefully make acceptance easier. In Thailand, the engagement is the biggest celebration regarding marriage and the wedding itself a much more subdued affair.

My son and the children visit Thailand again for a simple wedding ceremony which takes place in an office. So, I now have a second Asian daughter-in-law. I doubt there are many mothers of twice married sons who have not been present at either wedding, but at least I've never had to purchase expensive outfits or wear a frivolous hat.

His new wife will be leaving her job, saying goodbye to her family and friends and returning to England in the near future to join our little family. I'm hoping my son will now have a supportive, genuine partner and less stress with someone to share responsibilities. As far as I can ascertain the children are accepting and fond of the new addition to the family and I have everything crossed for the future of them all. I know things can never be perfect and I will have to put any concerns aside to allow them to move forward.

Unfortunately, little progress has been made with their mother and the visits to see her more sporadic. We have not made it difficult for her but she seems disinclined to set up regular meetings. It's not ideal when she cancels or alters arrangements and eventually she decides she doesn't want to see them again for several months, giving no reason. Although she maintains intermittent communication with them she rarely asks to see them.

On occasion, abuse, including death threats, are sent to myself, as well as horrible accusations and demands for huge amounts of money to anyone connected to my son. She seems to believe everyone owes her money from the past, when in truth she was always the one borrowing from anyone who would oblige. It's clear her state of mind is still disturbed and her erratic behaviour unchanged, so maybe it's best she doesn't see them. The welfare and safety of the children has to be top priority.

Time moves on and the plans for the newlyweds and the decision as to when the children will see their mother again are soon taken out of our hands in a way few could ever have predicted.

What About Now

May 2022

The past few years have been a strange time for everyone, in every part of the world, and maybe we should put our own petty concerns to one side when a global pandemic alters our everyday life in so many ways. But we are only human and situations like this are reminders that there is so much we cannot control in life. I guess that's one thing my personal experiences have taught me and I take nothing for granted.

From the painful decline and loss of my parents and husband to the deep seated fear that my son's marriage stood little chance of survival becoming a reality, in the main I have only been able to stand by and observe. I hope I have helped where I can, been a support through the most difficult times and made a little difference to the lives of my loved ones, but on the whole most events have been beyond mine or anyone else's control.

Life for myself and my family has changed dramatically but thankfully is mainly calmer and more settled. My son has done well to hold down a good job , run a home and cope with three children as a single parent for several years. He has also lost a lot of weight and managed to reverse his diabetes. After his second wedding overseas, he was eagerly awaiting the arrival of his new wife from Thailand. This time we were lucky, as her flight was one of few that were not cancelled due the spread of the virus.

At the start of the first lockdown a lone Thai lady arrived at Heathrow airport to start a new life in the U.K with my son and children. Restrictions were making life troublesome for everyone, but it occurred to me that if this new relationship could survive such a testing time, then the signs were positive. It has indeed survived; his new wife has settled well and enjoys living here. She's a talented, conscientious, industrious lady who appears to be able to tackle life from many angles; a tiny figure with a huge personality, a good sense of humour and mothering skills. I will never be one hundred per cent certain, but I dare to hope this relationship will really work out. Sometimes I witness traits I don't like, hear conversations that concern me and see some similarities to his first wife but it is not my place to judge or interfere. Experience has made me cautious and rather cynical but if my son is settled and content then that is as much as I can ask. Maybe it's the happy ending they all deserve at long last, but only time will tell.

The children have done amazingly well in my opinion. They have been through an awful lot and their young lives disrupted by one trauma after another. There are times of disharmony, tantrums, worry and concerns of course, but that is part of raising children whatever the circumstances. They are all very bright, independent and loving. Two of them are teenagers now which amazes me on a daily basis and I have everything crossed they will all find suitable paths in life and find the happiness they are entitled to.

Unfortunately, things have not improved a great deal with their mother, who still appears to be suffering from paranoia and displays some disturbing behaviour and ideas. The children have not seen her for over three years now, though she does phone and text them. I fear the youngest may completely forget her and the older two may become more distanced if she doesn't improve. There is little we can do about the situation, and sadly because of her actions we have had to ignore or block her on social media due to her sporadic abusive texts and death threats. Her contact with her children is erratic and often nonsensical. Statements about her relationship with the famous actor, her claims that everyone she has ever been in contact with owes her phenomenal amounts of money, her cult like declarations and philosophies on social media which are obviously not her own words all point to the belief she is not at all mentally well. We have no idea how she lives her life, who she associates with, what her plans are, if any services are involved with her, but it is out of our control and our priority is to ensure the children are kept safe and living in as stable an environment as possible.

She has sent some appalling texts and voice messages including death threats to me using several different identities and I have no choice but to block each one. For some reason she is obsessed by the idea I am performing black magic and witchcraft on her and others. If I was capable of such a thing I'd certainly be using my powers to help her recover, in order to be a decent mother to her estranged children, as despite everything I wish her no harm and would prefer the children to have a relationship with her.

On one occasion she turned up in a taxi at my house, totally out of the blue, and I was deeply shocked and upset. I had no choice but to wave her away, draw the curtains and call my son. Because of the death threats the police had to be involved, but I decided against pressing any charges as I felt it would just make matters worse. I can't seriously believe she would follow through any of her threats, but there's always a tiny element of doubt. When I saw her smiling through my window it was a shock, yet I felt sad that there is no way I can ever engage with her again, sad remembering the better times in our relationship and sad that she seems unable to approach the situation in a way that would benefit herself and her children. I still hope a time will come when she can.

As for myself, I try to take one day at a time and appreciate the positives. Living alone isn't ideal and often lonely, but there are advantages. For the first time I am free of responsibilities, restrictions and putting other's needs before my own, yet that is still an unfamiliar feeling. Solitary confinement is a punishment in some instances and sometimes it feels that way, but I work hard at keeping busy and involved as much as I can. I have some wonderful friends, both male and female, and I enjoy being with my little family now. I still miss my parents and my husband on a daily basis and I'm sorry the relationship with my stepdaughter and her family is irreparable, but that is her choice, not mine. My son's first wife has made inclusion impossible, but that is not my preference either. It doesn't console me a great deal and the hurts will never heal, but I know, as with most things in life, acceptance is the only way forward. I cry at the television programmes helping people find long, lost family when my own have just walked away and estranged themselves. I wish those things hadn't happened.

I try not to dwell on bad memories, even though they frequently invade my thoughts. I once had a dream in which I visited a hairdresser who proceeded to take off the top of my head and tidy it up inside and I don't think it takes an expert to analyse that. I certainly wish it was a possibility. I'm a bit of a neat freak and can only assume my habit of organising, rearranging and tidying drawers and cupboards is because it's something I can control, unlike what goes on inside my head. I've heard it said one of the greatest gifts of the human mind is the ability to choose what it thinks, but I don't seem to have that ability. There are no organised compartments inside my head; just a tangle of memories, flashbacks, anxieties, complexes, unfinished conversations and dark thoughts mingling with the mundane, and always accompanied by some musical ear worm that often takes days to burrow its way out, allowing the next one to wriggle in. If only there was an option to remove my head at night and replace it the next day when I feel ready to cope with it. If my body was half as active as my brain I'd be able to win marathons on a daily basis.

I admit it is still hard to keep going sometimes and I don't like contemplating the future. Depression still terrifies me and I am very aware it will most probably take me down again at some stage, particularly as my worst episodes are triggered by life events and we all know things we have always dreaded will most likely happen. But I have also learned we cannot predict the future and frequently the things we are convinced will cripple us emotionally are not the ones we've anticipated. Life is fragile and fleeting and mostly out of our control so the best we can do is surround ourselves with good people and do our best.

I hope I never have to return to a psychiatric ward, yet no longer dismiss the possibility. I often tread a fine line and have days when I don't cope well and question my state of mind. But each day I practice the methods that work for me. Life has to be worked at and sometimes that means doing what is right for me, though it may not be for others. I have learned sometimes being selfish doesn't mean to be wrong.

I'm thankful to cope and grateful I have avoided any more episodes of deep depression up to yet. I will always suffer from depression and I have reluctantly learned to accept that, difficult as it is. If others dislike me for my negativity, my dark thoughts and cynical views, then I have to accept that too.

I wish I was braver, optimistic, capable, confident and tough. I wish I could start each day with enthusiasm and hope and end each day with a feeling of contentment, followed by peaceful, restorative sleep. But that has never been the case and never will be. Whether it is our nature or life events that determine our character I don't know but I suspect it's a mixture of both. As we mature and develop understanding we know there will be life experiences that are difficult and painful, yet until they happen we cannot accurately predict how we will react or what effect events will have on our mental state. As a result, none of us can be sure that at some stage we won't suffer from a mental health problem. Yet, I still often feel inferior in many ways and have always had low self esteem, so all I can do is try my best to be the best person I can, warts and all. I try to work at believing I am no less than anyone else because I hurt sometimes, though I wish I was better at handling that hurt.

Let It Be

Afterthoughts

August 2023

Nothing ever has or ever will be perfect in life and none of us can escape trauma, disruption, loss and heartache. My own may be more or less than others depending on your perspective, but I feel my story needed to be told. I've lost count how many times I've started it then given up, how many ways of approaching it I've attempted and how many times I've edited it, for better or worse. Time marches on and I have reached the point where even though I know there is still room for improvement, the ultimate aim of having my book published has to be now. So, I apologise for any mistakes, repetitions, boring waffle, wasted words and anything else that may have irritated readers. I hope I have learned from my experiences and the efforts of writing about it all, and I hope others may learn something from reading it or at the very least take time to contemplate.

The telling of my story has been extremely difficult and at times frustrating but also a cathartic experience in some ways. It's been an impossible task to include every incident but I hope the difficulties of life events has been clearly evident. I'm sorry if it seems to be a story full of doom and gloom, but the true events I focus on are the very reasons I needed to write. Initially it was to be a story of my son's bizarre marriage, but at that time I hadn't anticipated a full blown breakdown lay ahead of me, so more and more as time moved on, the focus on mental health seemed the way to go.

I wish my story was different; upbeat, inspirational and positive, but life has not been that way for me, or so it seems. Whether it's because of events, my own perceptions or a combination I don't know, but as a reader I hope the story has at least made you think.

Everyone faces difficult times, some more than others, and the way we react to situations, trauma and relationships differs a great deal, but those of us who tend to break easily are most likely to suffer with mental health issues. We may make our own choices in life, but our innate nature isn't easy to alter, which I believe makes the most sensitive people more vulnerable.

I have always had melancholic and depressive episodes and am easily upset by personal events as well as worldwide incidents. I have many memories from my past, both good and bad but most are vague and misty. The period covered in this book, from my first major breakdown to present day seems a lot more vivid and intensely painful. I guess as we age, we experience a lot more serious and painful events and we cannot avoid loss, illness and death. Of course I have had some wonderful times amongst all the traumatic events, though many are now bitter sweet; treasured memories tinged with sadness.

Other people matter a great deal to me and I'm grateful to family, friends old and new who give of their time and offer support. I won't mention names of those I have learned to love through the real world and the internet, just as I have named no one in my story. You know who you are and I hope you know how glad I am to have you in my life, be it in reality or virtually. When I moved to my new home I was adamant I would change everything about my previous life and avoid familiar activities like joining a writing group. Within a few months I joined a writing group, but it is through the group I have made new friends and received the encouragement, support and help I needed to complete this book. I can never thank those people enough.

I ponder frequently whether fate and destiny exist, if there are spirit guides somewhere watching over us, if the things we experience in life are deliberate in order for us to learn lessons. There is no proof of any of this, but contrariwise there's no evidence against these beliefs, so I think it best to hope there is.

During the latter years of my life I have been involved with geriatric care, dementia, hospitals, care homes, lifeline services, disability, social services, cultural differences, domestic abuse, police and judicial services, child protection, online abuse, divorce and bereavement. I believe all these areas need a lot more input and understanding and that our world would be a better place if enough money and dedicated, properly trained professionals were employed to ensure things can progress and improve.

But it is mental health that concerns me most; something I have had problems with for most of my life and have to work at on a daily basis. My own observations are purely based on personal experience and I'm perfectly aware others may have endured similar situations that have been handled differently. My criticisms do not generally lie with individuals but systems, restrictions, lack of staffing, funding and in many cases misunderstanding.

Depression is a condition which is still very much misunderstood and devalued. Mental health will always be a complex and diverse subject and I make no claims to be an expert or offer any miraculous cures or infallible advice. Those of us affected all suffer in individual ways, react differently, and need variable types of help. My experiences have made me very passionate about the way mental health is perceived, treated and understood. I still feel there's a stigma surrounding it and patients are often made to feel ashamed, weak and inferior. That is so wrong on so many levels.

Mental healthcare, as in other areas of the N.H.S. makes it very difficult for those involved to care or give the time needed to get to know patients and their problems. Patients are more often than not seen as unfortunate visitors who need to be ejected and moved on as soon as possible, regardless of whether they are ready or willing, or if they have somewhere to go. Hospitals are staffed by many who are desperately trying to help, yet likely struggling with their own problems, and others who sadly show little or no understanding or compassion. When I was hospitalised I didn't know I would get better. But looking back, I can see I was definitely luckier than most of the other patients I met. Recovery shouldn't depend on luck, but too often it does. Many patients who are discharged are not fixed, not better, not ready, but pushed out the exit in order to make space for someone regarded slightly more in need. Many of these patients will keep on returning over time.

Sadly, we all know the funding and workforce both need increasing dramatically in many areas of healthcare. People suffering with severe mental health symptoms can't handle being added to ever growing waiting lists, can't cope with life until it's their turn and can't carry on without help. Unfortunately, this is a common predicament in these times and I wonder how many lives have been lost because of delay.

Medication may help some but there is far more to treating mental illness than prescribing pills to swallow. Yet frequently there is little else available, apart from the occasional counsellor and volunteers doing their best to provide distracting activities, and generally failing. Far more could and should be in place to help each individual patient with very differing symptoms and needs. We need those who refuse to give up on people working alongside those who have given up on themselves. Gentle handling is far less likely to lead to more breakages. We need assurance it's not a bad thing to be fragile, to be human, to make mistakes and admit them.

I have always been passionate about animals and their welfare and hate to see anything or anyone in pain or suffering, either physically or mentally. If there's one thing I think my life and experiences have taught me it is to always attempt to be compassionate, not to judge indiscriminately and to walk a mile in another's shoes before jumping to any conclusions.

I believe it to be an unusual and often traumatic road I have travelled with many a deep pothole and several wrong turns. I have endured many collisions and a couple of complete breakdowns, but I am still travelling, albeit at a slower speed with irreparable dents, and for this I am grateful.

It has been difficult to express my story through words and I am aware I digress, take scenic routes and unplanned twists and turns. My first infant school teacher told my mother I would one day write a book. I have started several and then enthusiasm, distractions and life have halted their progress. But finally, at a very late stage in life I hope to hold the book I have worked hard to complete in my hands. It may not be the book I wanted to write, more a case of needed to. My life may have presented many challenges, and like nailing jelly to the ceiling, they have been impossible to handle successfully, but now, when I thought finishing this book would be just another impossibility I am pleased to put these last words into place. For those who suffer from depression I hope you will empathise and gain something from my story and for those who don't, I hope it will help you to understand and offer support to those of us who do.

ANOTHER SMALL PRESS

A selection of titles available from www.anothersmallpress.net

Martin Costello

ALL THE THINGS I WROTE BEFORE I WROTE THE THING I ALWAYS WANTED TO WRITE

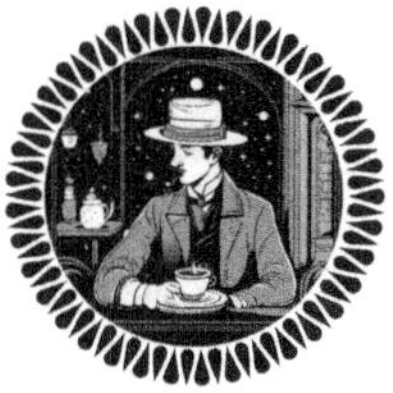

Eight picaresque ballads of life in the East Midlands - and sometimes on the seashore - by mild mannered anarchist & writer Martin Costello.

The elder boys carried the old sofa to the end of the pier, and the family set it up looking outward across the water so that they might catch an early sight of the ferry. They took turns on the watch through the long late afternoon, the children happily amusing themselves on the pier, under the pier, behind the sofa, in the mud, in the shallows, in the empty car park, on the roof of the ticket hut, up and down the ferry lane, along the grassy dunes of the strand, on the smooth round rocks of the tide wall and around the skirts of the mother Bidna to her passing amusement and then impatience and then amusement again. As evening threatened, a dog-walker from the lane helpfully called out that there would be no ferries that day, on account of the coming storm.

The story the author had always been trying to write is not included in this collection but happily is now complete after 22 years of editing.

£7.99

Adrian Bean

WHAT HAPPENED

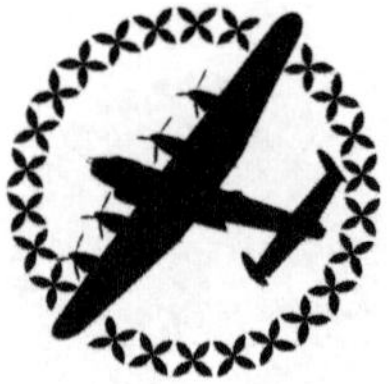

'RAF Syerston - that's where your uncle George's brother died during the war.'
'What happened?'
'I don't know...'

A short but intriguing conversation about a relative who died in a wartime plane crash started Adrian Bean on a journey that would obsess him for nearly two years. Curiosity, as well as a fascination with aeroplanes and the Second World War drove him to ask who was this relative and why had he never known of his existence? How did he die, and why? And what was the link with a wartime RAF bomber station and the Polish bomber crews who flew from there?

He would also come to ask deeper questions, not just about what happened in June 1941 but more recently, about the break-up of his own family, and just what it was that was driving him to find answers.

Sometimes funny, often disturbing, always honest, What Happened is a book about loss, and acceptance, not only in wartime; it is about discovery and memory and how we create and tell stories about the past to make sense of our own present.

£9.99

Roger Stennett

CLOUD CUCKOO LAND

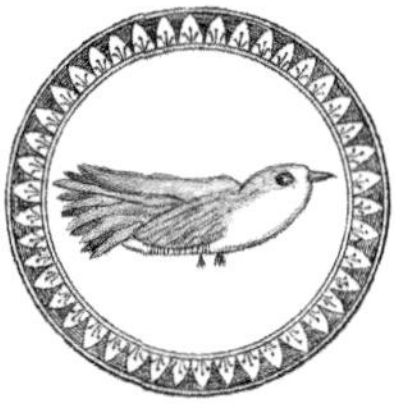

Roger Stennett is a Welsh poet, dramatist, screenwriter, audio and animation writer who has written thousands of poems since the 2020 global pandemic struck. Cloud Cuckoo Land represents the distillation of some 4,000 works into a selection of 100.

In a Classical Greek comic play by Aristophanes called 'The Birds', cuckoos were challenged to build a city in the sky amongst the clouds, to prove how powerful and godlike they were. Such a bizarre undertaking was clearly unreasonable and impractical, and ever since that time the phrase has been regarded as shorthand for impossible plans, unrealistic schemes and crazy dreams.

Classicist Roger Stennett remains undeterred.

Covering a wide range of themes and approaches including love poems, nature poems, historical poems, theatrical poems and poems of childhood, every page turn is an encounter with a new joy, an old friend, a common foe or a familiar sense of the cycles of lived experience.

£9.99

Printed in Great Britain
by Amazon

55978081R00101